Is Anyone Listening?

Domestic violence is in the public eye as never before, but how often are abused women consulted or involved in the new services and policies? This book investigates and reveals that the voices of survivors of domestic violence are often simply not heard; silenced, the women themselves become invisible.

Is Anyone Listening? draws on the experiences of other service user movements to provide a strong conceptual framework for thinking about abused women's participation in policy and service development. It discusses empowerment issues and the women's movement against gender violence, exploring how far refuge organisations and other women's movement services have influenced statutory services and vice versa. It includes many practical ideas for involving abused women in the improvement of both policy and practice, and gives examples of inspiring and innovatory projects.

Based on a study carried out as part of the Economic and Social Research Council's Violence Research Programme, *Is Anyone Listening?* offers a unique analysis of the sensitive and complex issues involved in developing service user participation within the domestic violence field. The insights it provides will enable policy-makers, activists, students, practitioners and women who have experienced domestic violence to move forward together.

Gill Hague is Senior Research Fellow in the School for Policy Studies at the University of Bristol and a fou   of the Domestic Violence Research Group   **ender** is Professor of Social Work and I   dy of Safety and Wellbeing at the Uni   **Aris,** formerly a Research Fellow at the   Seni Research and Evaluation Officer at

Is Anyone Listening?

Accountability and women survivors of domestic violence

Gill Hague, Audrey Mullender and Rosemary Aris

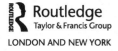
Routledge
Taylor & Francis Group

LONDON AND NEW YORK

First published 2003
by Routledge
2 Park Square, Milton Park, Abingdon, Oxon, OX14 4RN

Simultaneously published in the USA and Canada
by Routledge
270 Madison Ave, New York NY 10016

Routledge is an imprint of the Taylor & Francis Group

Transferred to Digital Printing 2009

© 2003 Gill Hague, Audrey Mullender and Rosemary Aris

Typeset in Times by
Florence Production Ltd, Stoodleigh, Devon

British Library Cataloguing in Publication Data
A catalogue record for this book is available from the British Library

Library of Congress Cataloging in Publication Data
A catalog record for this book has been requested

ISBN 0–415–25945–2 (hbk)
ISBN 0–415–25946–0 (pbk)

To Dorothy

How do they know what to do if they don't ask women in the situation? It doesn't make sense, does it? It's stupid if they go and set up things without women knowing about it and without asking women what they need, doesn't make any sense to me.

If they listen to us it is just so good. It makes the services better, just much better. No one has ever listened to us before. And then suddenly these posh organisations are. It brings tears to my eyes just thinking about it.

They are beginning to listen, they are beginning to try. That is the really big thing, isn't it, the fact that they are finally willing to at least *try*.

(Women survivors of domestic violence)

Contents

List of illustrations   ix
Acknowledgements   xi

1 Introduction   1

PART I
**Rethinking service user movements in relation
to women survivors of violence**   **5**

2 Women survivors of domestic violence as service users:
   the silenced group   7

3 The obstacles to empowerment: what kind of power
   for women?   26

PART 2
**Women's views and voices in domestic
violence services**   **41**

4 What abused women think of the services they receive   43

5 How much do agencies listen to domestic violence
   survivors?   58

PART 3
**How to engage in survivor participation and
consultation**   **75**

6 How to do it: empowerment and stigma   77

7 How to do it: policies, sensitivities and resources to make
   participation effective   89

8   Practical ways forward and innovation, including
    domestic violence survivors' forums   109

9   Further innovatory practice: Women's Aid, women's
    advocacy organisations and campaigns   125

10 Other methods of survivor participation and getting
    agencies to take action   131

11 Conclusion   145

EPILOGUE   **149**

    Words from women survivors of violence   151

    Womenspeak: a parliamentary Internet consultation
    with domestic violence survivors   160
    NICOLA HARWIN CBE, DIRECTOR, WOMEN'S AID FEDERATION
    OF ENGLAND

    Bibliography   163
    Index   174

Illustrations

Tables

5.1 Percentage of inter-agency forums and refuge services
     saying they involved service users   69

Boxes

7.1 Basic initial checklist   97
8.1 New and innovative practice in consultation with
     abused women   112

Acknowledgements

Many people have helped to make this book possible. First of all, we wish to thank all the many survivors of domestic violence who have talked and worked with us, and who have given us their time, energy, honesty and expertise, over our years of engaging in domestic violence work. Most particularly, our sincere gratitude goes to the women who had experienced domestic abuse whom we interviewed during the study on which this book is based. They assisted us, throughout, with the research and with ideas for this publication. Without them it could not have been written.

Very many thanks to Nicola Harwin, the Director of the Women's Aid Federation of England who was the consultant to the study and who has contributed a short section to the book. The study could not have been conducted without the dedicated work of our colleague, Wendy Dear, who participated in much of the research which forms the backdrop to everything we have written here. Our thanks to her and also to Hilary Abrahams who assisted with the research; to Ellen Malos who participated in the study initially; to Cassie Hague for administrative and research assistance; and, particularly, to Valerie Douglas who conducted secretarial work on the manuscript beyond the call of duty.

We are also most grateful to the many policy-makers, managers and workers in inter-agency forums, refuge organisations and statutory and voluntary sector agencies who agreed to participate in the study as interviewees and who assisted us to conduct the research in their areas. We are particularly grateful both to domestic violence survivors and to professionals who specifically assisted us in Coventry, the London Borough of Croydon and the North Somerset area (our main study areas), and in Sheffield and the Rhondda (our policy profile areas). In all of these areas, we were welcomed and assisted generously, particularly by the specialist domestic violence co-ordinators and the equality units and refuge organisations involved. In this context, we would particularly like to thank for their generous time and valuable ideas: Liz Blyth, then of the Coventry Domestic Violence Partnership; Angie Parks and the Coventry Haven project; Sobia Shaw of Panahghar; Maureen Storey of Sheffield Domestic Violence

Forum; Rohan Collier, formerly of the London Borough of Croydon Equalities Unit; and Pauline James of North Somerset Domestic Abuse Forum and North Somerset Action Against Domestic Violence. During the research, further small case studies were conducted with practitioners and policy-makers in the London Boroughs of Westminster and Newham and in Cleveland, to whom thanks are due. We also thank Welsh Women's Aid for their assistance and co-operation.

For welcome assistance with the book itself, our gratitude goes to the Hammersmith Standing Together Against Domestic Violence project, for input of ideas, to Voice for Change in Liverpool and the Phoenix Group in Westminster. Also, thank you to Sue Dzendera of Croydon Playcare, to Vicky Witherington, Croydon Welcare, and to Pat Francis and Lucy Darlow for contributing their words and expertise.

For commenting on drafts of this book, our thanks go most particularly for her extremely helpful contribution to Davina James-Hanman, Director, Greater London Domestic Violence Project. The text was also commented on most helpfully by: Vicky Grosser, Co-ordinator, Westminster Domestic Violence Forum; Norma Stoddard, Liverpool Domestic Violence Service Co-ordinator; Barbra Young, Croydon Domestic Violence Advocacy Project; and Hilary Abrahams and Ellen Malos, Domestic Violence Research Group.

Thanks also go to the advisory group for the study: Charlene Henry, Hadhari Nari Project, Derby; Jan Frances, Chair of the Women's Aid National Council; Pat Stafford, Nottingham Women's Aid Advice Group; Nadia Rush, Hammersmith Women's Aid; Ann Wardell, formerly of Cleveland Domestic Violence Forum; and Ann Harvey, Wiltshire NSPCC Domestic Violence Project.

On a personal level, during both the study and the writing of the book, we would like to thank, variously, Peter Burnham, Cassie and Keiran Hague and David Merrick for all their help, John Ashcroft for his love and support, and Dorothy Williamson, who died during the study, for her wisdom approaching death.

Chapter 1

Introduction

This is not just another book about domestic violence. Indeed, to learn about the detail of men's violence to women in intimate relationships – what it is, the damage it does to women's lives, what we can do about it – it will be necessary to look elsewhere. Over the last twenty years, a great array of books and other publications has been produced on the subject, furthering our knowledge and providing evidence and ideas to inform the way that society, governments and helping agencies respond (see, for example, Dobash and Dobash, 1992; Mullender, 1996; Hague and Malos, 1998). This, however, is a book with a different message. The message is about raising the voices of abused women themselves.

In this book, domestic violence is defined to mean violence between adults who are, or who have been, in an intimate or sexual relationship. We know that domestic violence has impacts on children witnessing or otherwise experiencing it (Mullender and Morley, 1994; Hester et al., 2000). We also know that it is a gendered phenomenon. While such violence can occur in gay and lesbian relationships and can be committed by women against men, the overwhelming majority of incidents are perpetrated against women, often by the men with whom they are most intimate (see Dobash and Dobash, 1992; Humphreys et al., 2000).

We have attempted here to pay attention to what women who have experienced domestic violence say and feel, especially if they have made use of service provision. However, we have also included a consideration of the views of abused women more generally. In the text, we often use the term, 'domestic violence survivor', because, even though many are severely victimised by the violence they have experienced, surviving is what all women try to do. We use the term as one of respect.

The argument which underpins this book is that it is necessary to reframe the way we think about the women who use domestic violence services and to see them as part of a service user movement, similar to other user movements which have lifted the voices of their members in recent years. Women experiencing abuse may be part of the women's activist movement against domestic violence, and are quite likely to have used services provided by it, but they have not generally been viewed as part of a service user group in their own right. One question which this book asks is why not. We will discuss how we can change both the practice and policies of agencies, and also the way that this issue is thought about in theoretical terms, so that abused women service users can be both heard and heeded. Thus, our arguments will be contextualised within theorising about user movements and new social movements more generally, and will then be developed in practical, concrete ways. The book looks at how much the voices and views of domestic violence survivors are currently seen as contributing to the policy process and goes on to illustrate ways in which these voices can be more effectively involved in service planning, provision and delivery.

One of the aims of movements of service users in general is to take control of how they are defined by others, notably by service providers, policy-makers and the general public. All of these movements are currently struggling to combat negative attitudes and labels, to be involved in key decisions which affect them, to decide for themselves what is in their own best interests, and to take action together to resist models of service delivery that may be oppressive or discriminatory, encouraging instead those that enable and empower (Barnes *et al.*, 1999). They also attempt to have some measure of direct control over the services they need to lead a full and rewarding life. One example concerns disabled people who have formed a powerful movement to argue for their rights. This movement has reframed thinking within society about disability to challenge a purely medical model in favour of an alternative social model and full citizenship for disabled people in every respect, as we will discuss further in Chapter 2.

The women's movement has similarly rethought and reframed issues in the specific context of discrimination against women and has, through the medium of feminism, changed almost everything about how we now view women. In the 2000s in the UK, very few people question women's right to work or to make choices about their own bodies and relationships. We can make a case that these basic arguments have been won after three decades of women's activism. Yet, women's everyday quality of life still leaves much to be desired and, in some respects, little seems to have changed at all. Gender violence remains a massive problem both in this country and across the globe, for example. In the UK, for an estimated one in three to one in four women (Mooney, 2000), violence is, at some stage, a part of their everyday lives and for many of them, as we shall see in Part 2, the services provided still do not meet their needs.

Above all, despite very serious efforts over many years in both the voluntary and statutory sectors, women who have experienced abuse and accessed services as a result, still do not feel safe. If services do not assist abused women to safety, one wonders what they do achieve. Further, survivors of domestic violence frequently do not feel able to speak freely about their experiences. They may feel blamed, silenced and stereotyped and, far from being seen as having expertise derived from what they have gone through, they are often blocked from full participation in service delivery as volunteers or as paid workers because they are seen as 'still in the experience'. On the plus side, there are some examples of very good, participatory services, women's projects and domestic violence multi-agency forums with well-developed models of user involvement, and we will explore these in more detail in Part 3.

The material for this book is drawn chiefly from a project, one of twenty within the Economic and Social Research Council-funded Violence Research Programme. This project, named 'Abused Women's Perspectives: Responsiveness and Accountability of Domestic Violence and Inter-agency Initiatives',[1] was conducted by the authors and by Wendy Dear, and was supplemented by knowledge from other research and from direct involvement with abused women. The multi-method study we conducted surveyed agencies and domestic violence forums on a national basis and also sought the first-hand views of domestic violence survivors. We will discuss, in the chapters that follow, the perceptions and opinions of the survivors we consulted about the direct services which they had received, as provided by statutory agencies, by refuge and outreach organisations and by inter-agency domestic violence forums. There is also much to learn from what abused women have to say about domestic violence policy and practice on a general level.

Overall, then, the book asks some very serious questions:

- To what extent are the voices of women service users heard in domestic violence policy development and service delivery and in inter-agency forums?
- Are services, practice protocols and policies responsive to these voices and informed in any way by service users?
- To what degree are services actually accountable to domestic violence survivors?

The immediate answers to such questions do not appear to be very encouraging. When asked to throw light on these rather hidden issues, one woman who had experienced domestic violence had this to say:

> We have no influence in their decisions. Not *really*, just pretend! The agencies pretend!

Arguably, unless the above questions can be answered in a positive way, services risk doing more harm than good, and could even place abused women in greater danger since only they can know in detail what will help them to be safe. If we fail to listen, we may fail to be of help.

Thus, this book is about the voices and views of domestic violence survivors and about the need for these voices to be heard – and, more importantly, responded to – by professionals. If the negative view expressed by the woman quoted above is typical of other women's experiences, how can agencies in both the statutory and voluntary sectors improve their provision and make themselves more accountable to those to whom they offer services?

Nothing in this book should be taken as a criticism of, or detraction from, the huge achievements of Women's Aid and of a host of other women's organisations in the UK. The record of the Women's Aid Federation of England, for example, which co-ordinates and supports over 250 local domestic violence projects in England providing over 400 refuges, help-lines, outreach projects and advice centres, speaks for itself (Women's Aid, 2001–2). We should be proud of all that has been achieved by women's activism over the last thirty years. But there is room for improvement in any service and success can bring its own challenges (for example, dealing with the strictures imposed by accepting state funding (Barnes *et al.*, 1999: 47)). We will address some of these challenges in later chapters.

Under the impetus provided by the activist movement, many statutory agencies and inter-agency forums also now take on the issue of men's violence against women in a committed way and a wide range of new policy and practice has developed across the board. These initiatives are often very helpful. However, they frequently fail to go far enough owing to shortage of resources, and they may have no mechanisms whatsoever in place for hearing what service users and other domestic violence survivors have to say. The ideas that we will offer will, we hope, help to make this more possible in the future.

Note

1   The study was supported by the Economic and Social Research Council, Award No. L133251017.

Part I

Rethinking service user movements in relation to women survivors of violence

Women survivors of domestic violence as service users

The silenced group

Women survivors of domestic violence have been users of dedicated, specialist services for thirty years in Britain. Yet, despite the burgeoning of policy, practice, and academic and political interest in user involvement in general and the long history of women's activism around violence, it appears that the voices of women survivors of domestic violence have been strangely silent in the context both of demands and of acknowledgement that service users should be consulted and involved. This chapter and the next will consider this contradiction from a theoretical perspective, explore how it has come about and what it implies, and, with an eye to the pros and cons, make suggestions for reconceptualising women as users of domestic violence services. Later chapters will look at practical ways of moving forward in giving abused women a more effective voice in service design and delivery than is presently available to them.

We begin by considering women's early organising in a wave of activism that has been seen as one of the first new social movements and a forerunner of service user movements.

Women's early activism

Women's activism constituted one of the earliest of the 'protest movements' that originated in the latter half of the twentieth century. The Women's Liberation Movement (known popularly at the time as 'the women's movement' or somewhat derogatively as 'Women's Lib', and in scholarly literature nowadays as 'second-wave feminism'[1]) flourished in almost every Western nation, and in many non-Western ones, in the 1960s and the 1970s (Coote and Campbell, 1987; Gelb, 1990). This coming together of women to make key demands for major changes in their role and status in society occurred at a time of broader social unrest, when civil rights were being pursued by African Americans, when the anti-Vietnam War protests were at their height and when students and workers took to the streets. Socialism, feminism and a broader struggle for democracy and social justice were in the air (see summaries, focused on women's struggles, in Coote and Campbell, 1987; Gelb, 1990; Dobash and Dobash, 1992; see also McIntosh, 1996 for a social policy analysis).

Out of this ideological background, women arrived at some very practical, emancipatory goals, and always regarded these as more important than ideas alone. Those who were operating from an equal rights (liberal feminist) perspective and some socialist feminists who saw gender as particularly connected to wider class exploitation, made real headway over the years in relation to equal pay, sex discrimination at work and fairer treatment in related areas of benefits and services. On the other hand, women who stood for a more radical, liberation agenda, including those who defined themselves as radical or revolutionary feminists or as socialist feminists, felt, and still feel, that there is a long way yet to go. This extensive range of women of different backgrounds, who came together to pursue broader, anti-oppressive objectives – with a focus on consciousness-raising for women and an end to men's patriarchal domination in the home and in all areas of society. Women took collective action in order to become personally, financially and legally independent of men, they wanted control over their own bodies and minds, and they wanted more support with childcare and in the home. Now, women are equal citizens in the law, and birth control and abortion are more readily available, but they are still treated as sex objects in large sections of the media and still undertake the bulk of domestic chores, with access to affordable childcare still inadequate.

Running as a clear thread throughout the debating and campaigning of the formative years of the women's movement was the issue of violence against women. Early consciousness-raising groups discussed the impact of men's violence on their own lives, and on the lives of other women, and rapidly saw the need to establish refuges or safe houses ('shelters' in the US) to which abused women could escape. This was a revolutionary idea at the time. Although a few refuges had existed in the previous century (see Pleck, 1986; Hague and Malos, 1998), the publicly accepted account of the first modern women's refuge anywhere in the world was at Chiswick Women's Aid, established in 1972. Other refuges were, in fact, established in various cities at the same time (though they received less publicity) and, from then on, the movement expanded rapidly with much dedicated activity that continues to the present day. The US, Canada and other countries followed rapidly. The first shelter in North America was in Toronto, with others established very quickly, for example in Minnesota in 1973 and in many localities, including Boston, by 1974 (Dobash and Dobash, 1992; Hague *et al.*, 2001a). Within the UK, as public awareness spread of what women were suffering at the hands of male partners, the topic was taken up nationally and regarded as part of a wider issue of male power. A seventh demand, added at the National Women's Liberation Conference in 1978 to those formulated earlier, was:

Freedom from intimidation by threat or use of violence or sexual coercion, regardless of marital status; and an end to all laws, assumptions and institutions which perpetuate male dominance and men's aggression towards women.

(Coote and Campbell, 1987: 18)

Refuges were organised under the banner of Women's Aid and, by the mid 1970s, existed in most areas in Britain, usually run by women's collectives (Hague and Malos, 1998). In 1974, they were organised into the National Women's Aid Federation. In keeping with the wider spirit of emancipation and egalitarianism that was prevalent at the time, the same conference that established the Federation saw it split from Erin Pizzey and her Chiswick colleagues because the latter wanted to maintain centralised control. Though both groupings have moved on in significant ways, the dual heritage remains, in the shape of the Women's Aid Federation of England and the equivalent organisations of Scottish Women's Aid, Welsh Women's Aid and Northern Ireland Women's Aid, on the one hand, and the organisation called Refuge, still operating from Chiswick but claiming a national role, on the other. The national Women's Aid federations exist to foster, promote and develop the refuge, outreach, aftercare and children's services that are offered by autonomous local groups, and to campaign, research, share information and promote public awareness of violence against women.

Thus one of the direct outcomes of the women's movement was the provision on a nationwide basis of services for women, designed and run by women, and conceptualised as meeting abused women's very particular needs. These have always been provided in the voluntary sector so that resources had to be campaigned and applied for from multiple sources that have never been secure. There is still no comprehensive acceptance of statutory responsibility for resourcing work with abused women since Supporting People goes only part of the way (see Chapter 4). Meanwhile, levels of male violence remain high, with one in every three or four women reporting that they have experienced it (Dominy and Radford, 1996; Mirrlees-Black, 1999; Mooney, 2000). Women's Aid's key asset is its thirty-year history – the depth of its roots. This does not mean, though, that there may not be elements of the work in women's organisations and related services that could be improved, and later chapters of this book will throw light on some areas where this may be the case if we continue listening to women's voices today.

The women's movement as a new social movement

As we saw above, Women's Liberation was one of the earliest protest movements. Thus, women have always been at the heart of what have now come to be called 'new social movements' (Dalton and Kuechler, 1990; Scott, 1990). These are social uprisings that are not dominated by traditional sources of friction; they are not about social class or people's relationship to the means of production, although some activists remain aware of, and engaged, in these issues. Rather, class is no longer simplistically dichotomised between the 'haves' and the 'have nots', while identity has ceased to derive solely from occupation (Charles, 2000). For women, this makes sense: it has always been possible to live with a wealthy man and yet to have no disposable income or personal freedom of one's own, or to hold down a well-paid job and yet to be harassed, abused and raped. Thus, class-based and job-based identity has never been the whole story for women. The new movements and pressure groups (Grant, 2000) engage in a personal, social and cultural politics that is sometimes more about collective consumption and purchasing power than about social class. Public protest and wide-scale direct action happen alongside campaigning by non-governmental organisations on environmental, identity and lifestyle issues and against racism and other oppressive systems, often replacing negotiation through elected representatives, membership of political parties and turnout at elections. Thus:

> citizens increasingly see themselves as consumers of public services and that single-issue interest groups offer the best way of articulating their specific demands.
>
> (Grant, 2002: 21)

There are many ways in which the women's movement from the 1970s onwards typified a new social movement. Women's goals have always been cultural as well as political, and are as concerned with the quality of life in civil society (equality, human rights, lifestyle politics) as with the economy and the state. They are 'transformative rather than redistributive' (Barnes and Bowl, 2001: 136). Women have also always sought change through non-violent action, consciousness-raising, networking, campaigning and so on, rather than solely through party or class politics or, for many, through any formal engagement with the party political process. Fitting its actions to its values, early feminism was marked by an interest in democratic and non-hierarchical organisational forms of all kinds, especially collectives: rotating responsibility for chairing and minuting meetings; giving everyone present an equal right to be heard; and sharing all work and decisions (Freeman, 1972–3). These principles were evident in the first Women's Aid groups and in refuge organisation, for example.

Women's activism has extended particularly widely throughout society because such disparate groups of women have been involved (Charles, 2000). Middle-class women, working-class women, students, minority ethnic women, housewives, unwaged and retired women have all taken action – not only for themselves but also for other causes such as peace (notably at Greenham Common), the environment and the struggles against racism and homophobia. This has involved the creation of new knowledge and new beliefs to challenge the old, questioning, and redrawing the parameters of what is considered political. Feminism classically did this and women across society continue to do it.

Women present, yet absent

Thus, women have been remarkably active and vocal in new social movements (NSM) generally – with the women's movement there from the beginning, and women consistently visible in all recent environmental, peace and other protests (as well as in more traditional trade union and class politics), in all of which they have worked tirelessly. However, the female contribution remains heavily under-represented in theoretical treatments, apart from those produced by feminist scholars themselves. As Charles (2000) notes, women's place and changing gender relations in the movements have been inadequately explored in the theoretical NSM literature, and there is little theorising of second-wave feminism as a social movement by scholars located outside it.

In critiquing this situation, Eschle (2001) reconstructs feminist ideas within theories about the cauldron of globalisation and ideas about 'engendering' global democracy through social movements. She explores both the strengths and the possible weaknesses of feminist approaches within a complex analysis that also investigates NSM theory. Eschle points out that, while all of this remains a hugely contested area, many NSM theorists do not identify with feminism, even while frequently stressing its role as one of the important social movements of the late twentieth century (ibid.: 4–5). Where more comprehensive treatments do exist, they often cannot accommodate the insights of feminist thought because the social analysts involved have tended to adopt more conventional approaches to enquiry. Nor does women's experience necessarily fit the theories very well, as Charles (2000) enumerates. Or should we say that the theories do not fit women's experience?

First, in Charles's account, women have not left economic issues behind, as new social movements are often theorised as doing. Women are disproportionately poor, are paid on average considerably less than men, and frequently do not live at the level of abstraction that can see the production of cultural signs as more important than material matters of production and reproduction (money and children!) in daily life. Women are concerned both with equalising or gaining political power and with lifestyle changes, hence they are both modern and postmodern and do not fit the 'malestream' theories very closely. (Perhaps the male theorists still have not noticed that the personal is political.) Second, within the realm of issue politics, feminist movements are not considered by all commentators to be new social movements. Second-wave feminism, by definition, cannot be new since it has continuity with the past.

Third, despite a very high participation rate by women in the new social movements themselves, there is little overt gender analysis in the literature on NSM, as noted above. The women concerned are of all age groups and occupy various relationships to the labour market, but there has been little scholarly enquiry as to who they are. Fourth, the theoretical field concerned (encompassing NSM and also resource mobilisation theory, RMT) is often not gendered and tends to assume a neutral and objective rationality that is commonly associated with white, middle-class Western males acting solely out of self-interest. Long-standing feminist critiques of instrumental rationality are largely overlooked, whereas people actually join social movements for a far wider range of reasons than pure self-interest or greed, again seeing that the personal is also political. Incentives may include values, friendship and other forms of solidarity, as well as, we might add, caring. However, doubting that participation would necessarily be in people's self-interest in reality, much RMT concentrates on looking at levels of resources and at leadership strategies required to encourage mobilisation (Baumgartner and Leech, 1998: 67–8, 75–7). Even though these theories are also used by feminist analysts themselves on occasion (Ryan, 1992), such an emphasis may overlook women and lead to a rather reductionist outcome (Eschle, 2001: 28).

Fifth, RMT, in a related point, tends to assume affluent Western forms of organisation as inevitable and most successful, and strategy as an organising principle. This has not been the historical experience of the women's movement, where collective organisation has predominated (at least until recently) and goals have often been pursued in a more instinctive, emotional way with democratic consensus and multi-tasking skills replacing top-down leadership and job specialisation. Finally, RMT is keen to measure success and failure, whereas a social movement may either succeed and become embedded or continue underground, and is likely to go through peaks and troughs, as we discuss in later chapters. Only hindsight can say what it really contributed.

All of these issues, though underplayed in the literature, are of particular relevance to abused women and their organisations. Women fleeing abuse are frequently on very low incomes, since, whatever their socioeconomic status before the violence, they commonly leave with nothing and have to start afresh. There is a historical continuity in the recognition of the needs of abused women that goes back to the nineteenth century and earlier (Freeman, 1979; Dobash and Dobash, 1981; Smith, 1989). There is enormous diversity within the collective action of abused women, since domestic violence is no respecter of class, creed or colour (Mooney, 2000). While there may be self-interest (and care for children) involved in seeking safety, there is also immense altruism for other women right across the refuge movement, including between refuge residents. Collective organisation does live on, though under threat, and there are certainly highs and lows in what it can achieve (see Chapter 6). Overall, we may decide to regard women's activism, including around violence, not so much as a new social movement but as an important 'contemporary social movement' (Charles, 2000), since it may not be brand new but it is still unquestionably with us.

From new social movements to user movements

New social movements are seen as the forerunners of service user movements. The activism of disabled people's and psychiatric survivors' movements, among others who use welfare services, has been remarkable in recent years. They have organised their own networks and campaigns, generated their own knowledge and theory and conceptualised their own alternatives to many aspects of social life, including health and welfare provision. They have voiced dual demands for user-run alternative provision, alongside claiming a voice within existing services. Disabled people and psychiatric service survivors have pursued a politics of social, cultural and political inclusion and participation, against a background of having been not just politically, but physically, excluded in welfare institutions and, even when living in the community, marginalised by 'discrimination, poverty and stigma' (Beresford, 1997: 4). Consequently, many see them as constituting a new social movement in their own right (Oliver, 1990).

A key reason why the user movements operate largely outside organised politics is that they are committed to individual participation, self-advocacy, self-organisation, finding one's own voice, speaking out and taking collective action through means such as mass protests and community arts, believing that these methods are likely to be more participative, more transformative of social attitudes and, quite simply, more effective (Beresford, 1997). In relation to disability, Oliver (1990) charts this distancing (or marginalisation) from traditional politics, along with the link between the personal and the political, the move beyond class-based, material demands and the international spread of the movement, as establishing the right of disabled people's self-organisation to be counted as a new social movement. Not all disabled commentators would agree. Shakespeare (1993) questions whether the label of 'new social movement' can usefully encompass both civil rights and liberation politics, considers that it ignores the continuity with disabled people's self-organisation in the past, and argues that (like the women's movement) the disability movement is grounded in identity, whereas peace and environmental activism are based on a shared interest – anyone can join (Shakespeare, 1993; see also Barnes and Bowl, 2001). Croft and Beresford (1996) summarise arguments that there is a lost opportunity for shared action around class-based politics and that identities frequently overlap, for example for disabled women.

Whether we accept the term 'new social movement' or not, however, user groups can certainly be seen to have their political roots in 'the emancipatory movements around gender and "race" oppressions' (Williams, 1996: 75) that predated them and hence to have continued the raising of popular voices against monolithic tradition and influence.

Women absent from the recognised service user groups?

Whether or not they are regarded as new social movements, user groups have made their impact. In his many publications about service users, Peter Beresford lists the now widely recognised groups that can be viewed in this way. Though the groupings have gradually expanded in his writing over the years, they have never encompassed abused women, as the following quotes consistently confirm:

> In recent years, movements of disabled people, psychiatric survivors, older people, people with learning difficulties and other groups of [users of] health and welfare services have emerged in the UK, North America, Europe and the South.
>
> (Beresford, 1997: 1)

> Recent years . . . [have] witnessed the emergence of welfare service users . . . including those of disabled people, older people, mental health service users/survivors, people with learning difficulties, people living with HIV/AIDS, etc.
>
> (Beresford and Croft, 2001: 298)

> During the last 20–30 years, we have seen the emergence and growth of new movements of welfare service users: of older people, disabled people, mental health service users/survivors, people living with HIV/ AIDS, people with learning difficulties, looked after young people and so on.
>
> (Beresford, 2001: 496)

Women are noticeable by their absence from any of these lists, not because Beresford has ignored them, particularly, but because they do not feature in the normal discourse about service users and have not been accorded public services in their own right (Mullender, 1996). Braye comes a little nearer when she offers her listing: 'Whether in disability, older people's and mental health provision, or in services for children and their families, the practice of service planners and providers is, in principle at least, open to scrutiny and influence by service users' (2000: 9). Abused women would figure in this list via their children where there were acknowledged child welfare or child protection concerns (Mullender and Morley, 1994), but, again, not in respect of their own needs.

Inside other user movements, women are present but may struggle to be heard. Disabled women have written about the personal in the politics of disability, from a feminist perspective (Morris, 1991, 1996; Begum, 1992), and have sometimes organised separately in order to gain an equal voice with men and to ensure that their particular issues – such as harassment, abuse and exploitation – are thought about (Powerhouse, cited in Morris, 1994; Members of Women First, 2002). In the world of psychiatry, women have campaigned against a fundamentally sexist view of what constitutes a mentally healthy adult; they have highlighted the histories of abuse that may cause depression or mimic psychosis, and have worked to make women safe from abusive therapists and fellow patients on mixed wards. They have also campaigned for childcare facilities in psychiatric settings, for women-only provision in therapies, and for alternative remedies, groups and community-based projects designed to make women feel stronger and better about themselves, as a challenge to the accumulation of more pills, labels and stigma (see summary in Mullender, 1995). Older women have argued for the right to 'grow old disgracefully' (Hen Co-op, 1993, 1995), rather than being seen as sweet old ladies who are grateful for any help they receive and always good for a bit of babysitting. We may conclude, then, that raising the voices of women's groups and making women more visible in broader user movements, can only be to the good.

Resemblances between the aims of the women's movement and those of recognised service user movements

It would seem useful to explore to what extent women's demands coincide with those of the now recognised user groups. (Later in this chapter, we shall also consider what, if anything, separates them.) In all the writings about user movements, both general and specific to particular groups, it is possible to discern certain key principles (Mullender and Ward, 1991; see also Morris, 1994), a number of which are explored below and which do seem to hold good for women in general and abused women in particular, though none has yet been carried through completely into practice, as we shall see throughout this book.

Rejection of negative labels

It may seem like the emptiest kind of political correctness when user groups start quibbling with language, but the kind of discourse that is used to discuss who someone is, what they are like and why, what they can and cannot do and what they need from others makes a vast difference to the fundamental way we perceive and treat that person. For example, the revelation in the social model of disability (Oliver, 1990) that disability is part of normal life, not somehow inferior, and that it is the social environment, rather than physical or mental impairment, that is handicapping turned traditional thinking on its head.

Like other user groups, women continue to be defined by male-dominated society as 'other', as lacking something. Theories of 'learned helplessness' (Walker, 1977–8) and terminology that stresses a 'victim' status (Kelly *et al.*, 1996), mean that abused women continue to be viewed as dependent, just as they were probably treated during the abuse. Empowerment, confidence-building and awareness-raising have always been key aims of the refuge movement, so that women's individual and collective strengths move to the top of the agenda, and language is crucial in achieving this.

Gaining a voice

Speaking out, being one's own advocate or, where this is not possible, calling on citizen advocacy or collective self-advocacy to put over one's true opinions and preferences (as opposed to having a carer or a professional assuming they know what is best) is a fundamental aspect of the principles, process, goals and achievements of all user groups. Finding a voice is the first stage in voicing demands and calling for social change.

Since women have been arguing their cause since the 1960s (and before), one might assume that this battle had been won for abused women. Yet the next chapter will show that even groups that are most vocal on their own behalf are rarely accorded a real say in decision-making in policy or practice settings. Furthermore, the findings of our study, reported in later chapters, suggest that there is an unacknowledged tendency in some domestic violence services to engage in practice that aims to protect survivors but, paradoxically, sometimes acts to silence them. This silencing tendency, we will argue, can lead survivors to minimise the extent and nature of the abuse they endure and may discourage their participation in initiatives designed to assist them. Thus, gaining a voice, even thirty years after the needs of abused women began to be recognised, is still an issue for women who have experienced violence from partners and husbands.

Challenging the control of others over one's life

User groups have sought to establish user-controlled services wherever possible and, where not, to make service planners, commissioners and providers accountable to service users for decisions and quality assurance.

Only by changing the way that service planners and providers think about users will we fit the services to the users, not the users to the services. This goes beyond the familiar debate within social care about making services needs-led rather than resources-led, because it is also about choice, not merely what a professional says the individual needs. This idea lies at the heart of user-centred services (User-Centred Services Group, 1993), regardless of whether or not they are user-run.

For women, taking control of one's own life and refusing to be the symbolic property of one's father or husband (with resonances, still, of the historical giving in marriage from one to the other as a chattel, to be owned, to obey unquestioningly and to have no voice in decisions) were fundamental aspects of what the women's movement demanded. Abused women have typically lived with men who have continued to believe in their own inherent superiority and right to rule the roost. It is often when women question such attitudes that they are abused. It is consequently particularly inappropriate if the services offered to women post separation from their abuser continue to seek to control their lives. User voices need to continue to be raised so as to ensure that women surviving men's abuse can make their own decisions and choices.

Generating theory

The first step in moving away from marginalisation and exclusion – in moving centre stage – is to have developed one's own analysis of the situation. The most notable example of this kind of reanalysis, not least because it has now itself become the norm in legislation and social policy (though not in medicine), is the social model of disability (see Oliver, 1990). This model recognises, as we have noted, that the major obstacles are situated outside the individual and that the challenge is for society, not the disabled person, to adapt and adjust. Priestley (1999) regards the analysis of a disabling society by disabled people as a 'counter-culture', throwing up new theory and new principles that have transformed policy and practice (though there is still some way to go). Service users 'have generated their own knowledges, theories and models, based on their first-hand experience' (Beresford and Croft, 2001: 295).

Equivalent theory generated right across the key fields of oppression in society by marginalised groups, according to Dullea and Mullender, includes:

- feminist theory and methodology;
- lesbian and queer theorizing;
- postcolonial and African-centred theorizing; . . .
- 'people first' and 'equal people' challenges to concepts of learning difficulties;

- child-centred research and theories of children's rights and perspectives;
- the challenges of the psychiatric survivors' movement;
- 'growing old disgracefully' ideas on ageing.

(Dullea and Mullender, 1999: 96–7)

Women, in generating a body of feminist theory, and also in rethinking
how new knowledge should be arrived at through research (Stanley and
Wise, 1983, 1993; Maynard and Purvis, 1994), have made an enormous
contribution to the sum of human knowledge. This is particularly true in
respect of men's violence, where all the key writers about women's and
children's experiences of domestic violence tend to be female and often
write from an overtly feminist position. Yet, paradoxically, this does not
necessarily mean that women's perspectives hold sway in respect of the
responses made to men's violence. In criminal and civil justice contexts,
for example, male-dominated discourses persist and, despite some improvements, it remains hard for women to see their partners appropriately
prosecuted or punished for the harm and fear they inflict (Edwards, 2001).
Women may own their own knowledge, but they have yet to see it acknowledged or implemented where it really matters.

Becoming empowered/empowerment

Empowerment means gaining personal strength and self-esteem, and then
social influence and power, typically through collective self-organisation,
through identifying with one another and through offering mutual support.
The following statement from the nationwide user-led disability project,
Shaping Our Lives, sums up the demands that arise:

> We want to be empowered as citizens and members of society and to
> achieve meaningful equality. Meaningful equality means having the
> same choices, opportunities, rights and responsibilities as all other
> members of society. It includes being enabled to live independently
> with the support that we require as a result of our impairments. Being
> empowered and independent means having full choice and control over
> the way we live. It is particularly important in relation to the provision
> of support services.

(Shaping Our Lives, undated)

With the exception of the phrase, 'as a result of our impairments', which
is specific to one user group, all of the above is true for women and reflects
the equality demands of the early women's movement. Whether abused
women have choice and control over the provision of support services, we
shall see in later chapters.

Differences between abused women and other user movements

At the same time, there are aspects of what abused women have to struggle against that are not as widely mentioned in the user group literature.

Confidentiality

Both exposure to danger and harm, and the resultant need for any responses to be grounded in issues of safety, security and confidentiality are fundamental in the field of domestic violence. In other fields, however, service use rarely involves life-and-death dangers, other than in the sense that some people would be unable to continue living without care. Confidentiality is rather rarely alluded to in relation to user rights. Interestingly, the other user group self-labelled as 'survivors', those of the psychiatric system, list it among key user rights that are denied in current services (Good Practices in Mental Health, cited in Harding and Beresford, 1996, as part of a consultation on service standards), thus establishing some commonality with abused women. Also, it is clear from other comments in the same publication that privacy regarding personal information is actually a concern of all groups who come into contact with social care services. It simply is less often mentioned, perhaps as a less urgent priority, but for abused women it can save lives.

Stigma/silencing

Women often feel unable to disclose that they are survivors of abuse. The stigma of sexual abuse, in particular, and of other types of personal violence means that some abused women still feel silenced (see Chapter 6). While stigma is a widespread experience among service user groups, it may perhaps be harder for abused women to raise their voices initially, since talking about their experiences may make them feel more, rather than less, ashamed. Over time, however, discovering that they are not alone in their experiences is a positive learning curve for women, as for other user groups.

Hidden among professionals

Survivors of domestic violence who are also professionals are often unable to disclose their experiences without losing credibility (as discussed throughout this book). This, again, is a shared experience with survivors of the psychiatric system and probably with other less visible service user categories. What may be different, however, is the widespread nature of woman abuse, and of child abuse, so that survivors are employed throughout the helping professions. Again, though, if we took a wide definition of mental distress, this might not be unique.

Overall, there seems no logical reason not to regard abused women service users as a user group with largely overlapping issues with other user groups, but with some areas of particular emphasis around confidentiality, safety, stigma and reluctance to disclose, all of which are experienced in common with at least one other heavily labelled group.

Why have women not been seen as service users?

So, if service user movements sprang from the earlier social movements, including gender activism, and if women are service users of specialist services, why are they not thought of as a service user group? Of course to become a viable social movement, self-organisation and campaigning are required and abused women service users have engaged in these to a limited extent so far. However, as we have argued, abused women can be seen as part of the wider activist movement against domestic violence which has been extremely vocal over many years, even though, in common with many user groups, it has often been ignored and overlooked. On a more general level, the huge social changes that have happened for women since the 1960s were never primarily about service use but about every aspect of women's lives. Indeed, the specialist services we now think of for women – refuges, rape crisis centres, women's community-based projects – had no forerunners that had to be transformed, as was the case for disabled people, psychiatric survivors and so on. The institution that women most typically wanted to transform was that of marriage (and the control of women's sexuality through it).

Perhaps even more significantly, abused women have had a constant battle to be accepted as entitled to a service from the statutory sector of welfare. In the social work arena for example, they were told until very recently that their difficulties were 'not a statutory responsibility' (Mullender, 1996), so it is not surprising that research has shown only about a third in non-refuge samples finding social workers helpful (McWilliams and McKiernan, 1993; Abrahams, 1994), with black women giving particularly negative feedback (Mama, 1996). Even now, most local authorities only prioritise cases that have a child protection aspect, typically where the abused woman is thought not to be able to keep the children safe – not surprisingly if she is given no help with her own life-and-death situation (Mullender and Morley, 1994). Studies have repeatedly revealed social workers' tendency to focus narrowly on the children, to the detriment of women's safety (Maynard, 1985; McWilliams and McKiernan, 1993; Humphreys, 2000) and sometimes of children's safety, because the danger to children from a man who abuses his partner is not recognised (Bridge Child Care Consultancy Service, 1991). This situation has only patchily improved since the overlaps became more widely accepted between the abuse of women and the abuse of children (Humphreys et al., 2000). Yet, in fact, local authorities are free to prioritise support for services for abused women and their children, through their Community Care Plans, Children's Services Plans and Crime and Disorder Strategies, which would work to keep both women and children far safer than at present (Mullender, 1996). Some are beginning to do so.

Because abused women have never been thought of as users of social work and other services in their own right, there has been no struggle to gain a user voice and hence, now that user views are being routinely sought in all sorts of government and local government initiatives, women are frequently omitted from consideration. We would argue that this is a serious gap and that the time has come to challenge it.

What could be gained from listening to women as service users?

User involvement is crucial in improving agency responses to any area of human need, and domestic violence is no exception. An adequate under-standing of the nature and scope of the problem requires that the myths about it be replaced with accounts of women's actual lived experience, since these constitute the most appropriate evidence on which to base professional intervention (Mullender, 1996). This is only likely to happen if women's stories are voiced and heard. Service providers, having been put into the role of experts, need:

> to understand the complexities of women's attempts to escape; the use by male partners of all forms of abuse to prevent this; the interaction between the emotional impact of the abuse and the difficulty of nego-tiating the maze of legal and welfare services; above all, the crucial need for advocacy, self-help and support services to empower women through this process on their own terms.
>
> (ibid.: 1)

This understanding can best be acquired from another kind of expert: that is, from the survivors of domestic violence themselves. The opportunity to share experiential knowledge between survivors through the self-help ethos of Women's Aid also provides women themselves with mutual access to an expert resource which is different from that available from health and social care professionals and which some women may consider more useful than professional input. Furthermore, the establishment of dialogue between users and providers of services creates forums in which experien-tial and professional knowledge can be shared and thus offers at least the possibility of transformation and change, as we shall show in later chapters.

There is another crucial reason why the voices of abused women must be heard. It is now widely recognised that it is essential to include partner reports as the most important measure of whether violent men have changed after attending a perpetrator programme (Mullender and Burton, 2001). This is because women partners and ex-partners routinely mention more incidents of abuse than do perpetrators themselves or than are contained in official records kept, for example, by the criminal justice system (since most domestic violence goes unreported and abusers tend to minimise and deny it). It is also important because women are the only ones who can say whether they are still living in fear, even if the actual violence has stopped. For example, in one major study in Scotland, three-quarters of women reported persistent pushing, grabbing and slapping, as against only one-fifth of male partners; women reported more, and more frequent, injuries, whereas perpetrators rated both their violence and the injuries they inflicted as less serious (Dobash et al., 2000). This is not usually because women are exaggerating what has happened to them. American research has shown that women tend to report what has occurred accurately, with accounts that remain consistent over time and in response to interrelated interview questions, together with evidence from hospital and arrest records to substantiate their stories (Gondolf, 1998). Consequently, we can say that women's voices are vital to efforts designed to change the behaviour and attitudes of the men who abuse them.

Though there can be obstacles (which will be explored in the next chapter), it is not impossible to achieve this open and honest dialogue with and between service users in any category. In recent years, a generic litera-ture on user involvement in service provision has developed, featuring 'how to do it' guides aimed at professionals, including those in local authorities who purchase (Lindow, 1994a) and commission services (Department of Health, 1996b). Key bodies established to work for these aims have included the User-Centred Services Group (1993), the Open Service Project (founded by Peter Beresford and Suzy Croft) and the National User Involvement Project, through which the Department of Health produced guides on involving service users as consultants and trainers (Department of Health, 1996a) and in commissioning services (Department of Health, 1996b). In the same year, the Department funded consultations on the standards service users and carers expect from social services (Harding and Beresford, 1996) and on involving them in local services (Harding and Oldman, 1996). Women need and deserve to be part of these debates.

What abused women lose by not being regarded as a user movement

The fact that abused women have never won the battle to be regarded as users of mainstream services in their own right, and are not regarded as a user movement, matters now because user voices and user viewpoints are being consulted more than ever before. Independent representation aimed at giving people a say and a choice in services has become a constant official refrain since the Citizen's Charter (Home Office, 1991). Advocacy is now enshrined in government policy, featuring, for example, in the Valuing People White Paper in the field of learning difficulty (Department of Health, 2001), in Quality Protects guidance, NHS reforms in the shape of Patient Advocacy and Liaison Services, and elsewhere. The role of advocacy has been recognised, too, in relation to the protection of vulnerable adults, both nationally (e.g. Law Commission, 1995) and locally (Bennett and Kingston, 1993).

Government is still working here largely within the consumerist model, supporting the marginalised individual to make his or her views known within a framework of national standards, rather than from a collective activism stance. Standards are imposed from the top down but it still matters that women are excluded. We live now with a politics of participation in social welfare (Beresford and Croft, 2001) which emphasises consumer feedback and which 'has given those movements whose members are users of welfare services an important space to push for their demands' (Williams, 1992). The Best Value Framework, for example, now requires consultation with service users and with local people more generally (see also Chapter 7). The issues of information and consumer choice must also feature in Community Care Plans and Health Improvement Programmes and, here, there *is* a collective element in that users' and carers' own organisations are among those consulted, with marginalised groups given special mention.

The newly established Social Care Institute for Excellence (SCIE) is including user-generated knowledge among the sources it will consult in recommending evidence-based best practice:

> Users' and carers' experience and expertise on what works, along with the experience of practitioners and of service providers, and the evidence from research and service reviews, should be an important part of the social care knowledge base.
>
> (Social Care Institute for Excellence, 2002: pages unnumbered)

If abused women are not among the users being consulted, then their knowledge – that they do not feel safe, that confidentiality is a life and death issue and so on – will be excluded from consideration. Yet, provided they are prepared to listen, social workers and other social care professionals are among those who can help women be safe or can place them in renewed danger. One classic study in this particular arena revealed that as many as one in three social work cases involved known instances of domestic violence (Maynard, 1985), and a similar figure appears if social workers are asked to estimate the prevalence of domestic violence in cases where children are on the child protection register (Hester and Pearson, 1998). This last number can double when practitioners more experienced in domestic violence matters look at the cases concerned (ibid.). If users are not listened to, services will march on unchanged, possibly colluding with – or even increasing – the dangers for women and children, or they will be 'improved' according to political or service provider whim and users will become yet more disenchanted.

Having a voice does not happen automatically. It takes effort, as this book will illustrate. So, if a particular group is not conceptualised as part of the body of users, its views will quite simply be overlooked. We are not making a naive or simplistic argument in calling for women who have experienced violence to be included among the service users who are routinely consulted. We are fully aware of the potential for tokenism and of the smokescreens that can obscure the lack of real change. The next chapter will explore in greater depth the obstacles to, and limitations involved in, user involvement in the design and delivery of services. However, being ignored – finding oneself outside looking in – is damaging both to service users and to practitioners, so this chapter has concentrated on arguing why abused women should be conceptualised as a service user movement and what could be gained from this.

Conclusion

Women have fought some tremendous social battles since the mid twentieth century and have won enormous social advances but they have never been able to count on anyone else to include them. Certainly, neither official thinking nor the user participation literature more widely has taken women on board as a user group to be consulted about service provision, any more than new social movement theorising has given them the place they deserve, despite women having had their own theory and their own user-run services for some decades. Abused women in particular tend to remain marginalised. Yet there is no logical reason why women domestic violence survivors should not feature in user arguments, demands and action. As we have shown in this chapter, the empowerment demands of the women's movement and of other user movements overlap almost entirely in terms of process (having a voice, winning rights and respect and so on), and, where abused women do have particular issues that affect them disproportionately, such as stigma and confidentiality, these are also shared with at least one other identifiable user group. Meanwhile, government policy has moved strongly towards user consultation and the provision of advocacy (at least within an individualised, consumerist model of user participation which will be explored in the next chapter), so that it is becoming increasingly worthwhile to be on the inside rather than the outside of the user movement. Also, if policy planning and service development lack abused women's voices, they will be at best flawed and incomplete and, at worst, dangerous.

We need to think of women service users as social actors, as socially included, not excluded. However, we can no longer see 'women' as a homogeneous group, or as a dichotomised or essential category. There is difference and diversity between women, and services must meet the needs of all, including the needs of children if women themselves become abusive (Mullender *et al.*, 2002). This means ensuring that all women are included, black and white, lesbian and straight, disabled and non-disabled. It means hearing the voices of women of different ages, women married and with children or not, and women of wide-ranging ethnicities and backgrounds. Service providers and policy-makers cannot afford to ignore these voices, as the rest of this book will illustrate.

The next chapter will show that all user groups and movements, including abused women, still face obstacles to real participation. The research reported in the later chapters of this book may, therefore, have much to offer to the service user movement across the board, and not just to abused women, in further exploring the obstacles to involvement and particularly in offering some possible remedies.

Note

1   What is now referred to as 'first-wave feminism' was the activism of the nine-teenth and early twentieth centuries that led up to women gaining the vote and to other advances.

Chapter 3

The obstacles to empowerment

What kind of power for women?

Following on from the argument we developed in the last chapter, we are not so naive as to assume that gaining a voice as a user group would leave abused women wholly better off. User participation has been widely critiqued as open to tokenism, co-option and exploitation. There needs to be a clear understanding of the dangers and limitations, and of action that can be taken to combat these, if women are to obtain full benefit from a new level of involvement. Indeed, our own research study (reported in later chapters) sought to distinguish between the mere semblance of involvement, on the one hand, and survivors of domestic violence exerting actual influence and decision-making power, on the other.

The problems with both the theory and practice of empowerment through user participation are well-documented (Croft and Beresford, 1996; Humphries, 1996; Ramcharan *et al.*, 1997). They revolve around issues such as competing ideals, professional vested interests and the demands of funders. In this chapter, we explore a range of barriers to empowerment, grouped under considerations of conflicting models, managerial and professional agendas, practical obstacles and contested understandings of power. All of these may prevent abused women, as well as other groups of service users, from having a full say in the policies and services they need to help them survive. In the chapters that follow, based on our research with women survivors of domestic abuse, we will see some of these obstacles operating in practice, as well as a number of effective ways round them, and we will conclude with some useful advice to those who want to be part of abused women gaining a real voice in refuge, multi-agency and statutory responses to men's violence.

Conflicting models: two approaches to empowerment

We saw in the last chapter how there can be a tension, even within the aims of user movements themselves, between concrete change and a broader philosophy of consciousness-raising and empowerment. At the wider, societal level, a fundamental element of the understanding required to give a real say to women (or to any other user group) is to perceive that there have always been two approaches to user empowerment (Mullender and Ward, 1991; Croft and Beresford, 1996; Forbes and Sashidharan, 1997). These can be broadly identified with individual consultation, on the one hand, versus finding a collective voice, on the other – what we might see as a continuum from user involvement in top-down policy and practice agendas to users' control of their own agendas. Over the same period that the theory and practice of empowerment were coming to the fore, in the form of a call for a full, anti-oppressive sharing of power with service users (e.g. Mullender and Ward, 1991), social policy in the Conservative era was introducing the ideas of the market into community care provision, and John Major's *Citizen's Charter* (Home Office, 1991) was arguing for individual choice.

The language of the two philosophies met in the middle, around words like 'choice' and even 'empowerment', but they have never used the terms to mean the same thing. The welfare consumerist model of the New Right (during the Thatcher era and subsequently) concerned the right for those who could afford it to buy choice, among whichever services survived the move to a mixed economy after comprehensive public provision came under attack. The user movement, on the other hand, had fundamentally different demands, calling for a full say in controlling decisions about what kinds of services should be provided, in what ways and to what standards – indeed, often for the right to run their own services (Mullender and Ward, 1991). Thus, it is always essential to be mindful of the continuum between 'consumerist' and 'democratic' models (Croft and Beresford, 1996: 186) and to be wary of what lies behind any general discussion of 'user participation' or 'user involvement'. The speaker may be situated at one extreme or the other of the continuum, or may simply never have thought through the issues.

The consumerist approach is usually associated with policy-makers, politicians and service providers, and its aim in offering users participation is really to make services more efficient, cost effective and responsive, rather than to redistribute power. Users are being 'used' to deliver this end. The democratic approach on the other hand, is associated with service users and their organisations, who are primarily concerned with participation as a way of improving their lives, winning rights and exercising choice and some control over the policy process. This can be summed up in the short-hand phrase: 'user empowerment'. Hence, as Croft and Beresford (1996) emphasise, participatory initiatives can be a route either to redistributing power or holding on to it. They call this 'the paradox of participation' (ibid.: 192) and, for them, the key to resolving it is being clear about the under-lying objectives – whether the initiators of the move to involve users see it as an emancipatory project (Leonard, 1997; Pease, 2002) or simply as a

means to a more efficient status quo. Both models do, to some extent, refor-
mulate the way we view service users, placing them far more in the centre
of services and giving them some kind of a voice, but it is important to
remember that the approaches diverge fundamentally around the question
of power, to which we shall return later in this chapter.

Losing hold to managerialist agendas: the encroachment of bureaucracy

Recognising this divergence, according to Croft and Beresford (1996),
helps us to understand why user participation 'is so often treated as a
rhetorical flourish rather than a serious policy and why it has become so
devalued' (ibid.: 192). Under New Labour, we have stayed largely with the
consumerist model, first introduced under Thatcherism. The modernisation
agenda that is currently being promoted is managerialist in many respects.
Users are consulted (classically in focus groups – has any other political
group ever been identified with its own research method?), but they are not
in charge. They are listened to, and possibly respected now by politicians
and the public more than are the public sector officers and social workers
who serve them (though this is not generally true for women users of
child care services), but they are not given control of budgets. (Direct
payments that are given to users to buy their own services are allocations,
not overall budget decisions.) Purchasing from preferred providers and
suppliers under block contracts has reduced the opportunities for users to
exercise choice (Dowson, 1997), rather than increasing them as the community care reforms were meant to do. Indeed, service providers may want
to involve users in order to improve efficiency and reduce costs rather than
to have them exerting any real influence or making changes. They may
co-opt users to give the impression of participation rather than genuinely
wanting to share or transfer power.

'Safe' ways to involve users, as far as service providers are concerned,
include using consultative procedures as delaying tactics, diverting users
into alternative agendas, legitimating decisions by having users present,
and inviting tokenistic individuals rather than talking to representative
groups of users (Croft and Beresford, 1996). All the talk of user participation and of a move to more user-centred services can be hijacked by
those whose chief interest is the effective management of budgetary allocations. For example, service users who receive a questionnaire asking
them to state where they prefer to access services, may find, if they reply
that it was handy to contact a social worker through the GP surgery
following an accident, that they are contributing to the closure of social
work offices elsewhere in the town that they might have found handier or
more appropriate for other kinds of problems (a real example). Service
users want to get involved, in order to have a say and to broaden the basis

of participation, not to be made party to a managerially-driven agenda, such as a reduction in service, which has never been fully explained.

In a similar vein, Anderson (1996) argues that '[t]hose with power-over will inevitably try to de-politicise by appropriation of the terms and definitions' of empowerment; those who hold the power may not openly oppose collective action but they diffuse it just as effectively by individualising it, or by employing its strategies 'in top-down, disempowering ways' (ibid.: 74). These and other forms of tokenism – giving the appearance without the reality of involvement – can be far harder for users to handle than outright opposition because they appear (and may actually be) well intentioned and because they buy off opposition with partial, incremental change that does not threaten the real location of power and influence. If these tactics are being used to mask, justify or sell policies that primarily aim to save money, cut back on services and shift blame, then we are driven back into questioning who holds the power and for whose benefit they are exercising it (as further discussed on pp. 34–9). The acceptance of funding for a user-run group or service, in particular, may have strings attached and can result in interference, especially from the more mainstream sources (Lindow, 1994). We found examples of this in our research, which we discuss in later chapters.

Who initiates participation: the professionalisation of empowerment

At the front line, there are also tensions between practitioners and service users. Through the 1990s, empowerment became a major focus and, indeed, an assessable requirement for qualified practice in the welfare professions. This was fought hard for by professionals who were committed to the issue and to anti-discriminatory policies. Paradoxically, though, a mainstreamed emphasis on empowerment can present a further problem if the professionals who 'do the empowering' (Baistow, 1994: 37) make 'claims to empowerment as a knowledge base' (Gillman, 1996: 108). This can place them, the professionals, rather than users, at the centre of the process – a position from which they may appropriate both the definition and the operation of empowering practice and once again assume the role of experts in determining other people's needs. This professionalisation of empowerment can be seen as a reaction to the threat to professional knowledge and expertise, and to professionally designed services, inherent in the development of new social movements and user groups that we outlined in the last chapter (Gillman, 1996).

There have been many examples of user-designed and user-led services that celebrate the knowledge and expertise of users in identifying and meeting their own needs (particularly well documented in relation to mental health (see, for example, Barker and Peck, 1987; Chamberlin, 1988; O'Hagan, 1993; Lindow, 1994)), as well as moves towards people taking control of their own health and welfare. These initiatives may be beneficial for service users but they can also threaten professionals who see their position as rooted in their exclusive rights to these areas of practice. So, while professional theories of empowerment might appear to be anti-discriminatory, they need to be treated with caution (Gillman, 1996), because, if empowerment is professional territory, there are dangers for those who seek to empower themselves, in their own ways, or who prefer not to be empowered by professionals at all (Baistow, 1994).

A particularly trenchant criticism of the notion of user empowerment is that the constant talk about it has been a 'substitute for action' and a 'comfortable delusion of change, while allowing professionals to keep their power in all the ways that matter' (Dowson, 1997: 101). Thus, the attention given to user empowerment may not signify any appreciable degree of professional commitment to hand over power or that any real progress has been made. Once again, Dowson sees the struggle for power taking place entirely on professional territory and regards status differentials, in this case between people with learning difficulties and the staff who work with them, as, to date, immune to change. Furthermore, although professionals can offer evidence of service users having been given a voice in all sorts of projects, consultations and advocacy groups, they typically still do not have power as tenants, consumers or employees, and being 'consulted' is simply not a substitute that the general public would readily accept in place of these other roles, he argues. 'When the initiative for user empowerment rests with people who would best serve their own interests by holding on to the power they already enjoy, there is good reason to be sceptical about the prospects for real change' (ibid., 1997: 107). In our study, the operation of power emerged repeatedly as a vital issue to address in terms of user participation by survivors of domestic abuse, as we will discuss in Part 3.

At a purely practical level, the lid can be kept on user dissatisfaction by professionals indulging in power games, linguistic subterfuge or a resort to procedures. In domestic violence services, multi-agency forums can become talking shops that fail to challenge inaction and consequently make little real progress (Hague et al., 1996). If they do engage in dialogue with service users, professionals may baulk at or dilute user involvement because they anticipate criticism, unrealistic demands or outright anger; it is hard to be open to complete rethinking of how one does one's job (Harding and Oldman, 1996). This kind of questioning is unfamiliar and uncomfortable for professionals, and may make them unduly defensive. It is especially hard to be challenged by patients and service users who have traditionally been labelled as vulnerable, or as unable to cope or make their own decisions (Barnes, 1999); that is, by people who are 'discredited' (Lindow, 1994: 5) and who have a 'spoiled identity' (Aris *et al.*, 2002, drawing on Goffman, 1963), as we discuss in detail in Chapter 6. Even more so, in organisations that have a high level of user involvement or are user-controlled, it is hard to face being hired and fired by service users. Professionals and their agencies are also suspicious of non-hierarchical forms of organisation (Lindow, 1994a). They tend to want to know who is 'in charge' and to mistrust the idea that collective action can mean collective management (and vice versa). Getting past all these negative assumptions and prejudices takes time and particular effort, as we shall see in later chapters.

Barriers to involvement

In practice, the process of participation may be far from smooth for service users. Formal consultative procedures can tend to become enmeshed in bureaucracy and administration, and levels of actual involvement may be uneven, resulting in only limited achievements. This may prove 'stressful, diversionary and unproductive' for service users unless adequate support and access provisions are put in place (Croft and Beresford, 2002: 388). Many studies of community, disability and user groups have confirmed this scepticism. Grant (1997), for example, records a parent saying that there did not seem much point in being consulted if the experts were going to take the final decisions, an issue that was frequently raised, too, by service users we interviewed in our own research.

Practical limitations

A range of practical obstacles are on record as likely to impede user participation. In a study of user involvement in community care, for example, Servian (1996) found that the actual process was disempowering, owing to management-controlled agendas and incomprehensible procedures, power structures that limited levels of participation, scarcity of resources and 'buck-passing'. Every attempt at empowerment by managers and frontline workers had its downside in the way it actually operated. Crucially, one carer even doubted whether the consultation forums in which users and carers participated were genuinely part of the decision-making process, since they seemed to keep the real issues from being aired. Grant (1997) lists shift work, lack of available transport, poor health and caring responsibilities as concrete barriers to getting involved. All of these can affect women disproportionately. Croft and Beresford argue for adequate support to make a reality of participation, 'on equal terms' (2002: 390). We shall see in Part 3 that this can mean training, mandating and practical matters like paying travel and childcare costs.

Psychological barriers

Not all the obstacles to user participation are essentially practical. Some are psychological. Despite the fact that all the survivors interviewed in a previous study of multi-agency work in relation to domestic violence thought that women's voices should be heard in their local domestic violence forum and that it was important that agencies should listen to and learn from women who have experienced domestic violence, some were less positive in relation to being personally involved (Hague *et al.*, 1996). Similarly, in a study of the All Wales Strategy for the Development of Services for Mentally Handicapped People (Welsh Office, 1983), Grant (1997) found that a typical response to the question of user partici-pation (in this case from a parent) was: 'Good idea but don't ask me; it requires people with particular qualities – people who can speak out, people with time, people whose expertise ... is acknowledged' (ibid.: 126). Thus, a lack of confidence can be a real barrier, which may need considerable support and encouragement to overcome. Grant found that a large number of people were unaware of their right to participate, or of the purpose of this, despite widespread publicity. And many of those who did get involved wondered whether the degree of change achieved made their own or others' participation worth the effort. We might assume that this could deter service users from being involved on further occasions.

Further disincentives to involvement are outlined by Harding and Oldman (1996). Users are not used to being listened to and may not believe that this can really happen. It may feel unsafe to speak out if you are depen-dent on others for their goodwill, help and practical resources, or if what you are likely to say feels confrontational because you need to tell agencies that their well-meaning efforts to date have been tokenistic or positively unhelpful. Certainly, some participants in Servian's study (1996) felt that speaking out and expressing their views might have been seen as aggres-sion, thus getting them into trouble. Service users might feel nervous, lacking in confidence and unable to participate on an equal basis with apparently powerful and articulate professionals (Harding and Oldman, 1996). Further, participation may not extend equally to everyone if some user group members lack the patience to help others speak out and instead do all the talking themselves (Adams, 1996).

There may also be issues of racism and of other types of discrimination and disadvantage coming into play. Black women may find it harder to speak out in front of white women, users in front of carers (and vice versa), and lesbian service users may have their own issues which it would be easier to share in a separately convened group, for example.

A gendered hierarchy of involvement?

From the above discussion, it is clear that those who would benefit most from change – the most powerless – frequently do not feel able to participate in the process (Wallerstein, 1992). Hence many women, and particularly abused women, are likely to be at a disadvantage. When women do decide to get involved, it may not be on an equal basis. In mixed community groups, they may contribute disproportionate time and energy, deriving less benefit at greater cost than other participants (Anderson, 1996). In community action contexts, there is some evidence that women are less likely than men to be paid for their efforts, less likely to be in leadership roles, more likely to take on the bulk of the detailed organisation, and more likely to be assumed to have the time for voluntary work (Anderson, 1996). Yet men are more likely to benefit from the gains that such campaigns may win, unless women organise separately to raise their own issues and to ensure that a diversity of women's views are heard within this (Dullea and Mullender, 1999). One reason why women have established their own groups and organisations is to ensure that their agendas, including decreasing men's violence, can be pursued.

Accusations of unrepresentativeness

Clearly, it is hard for any individual woman to speak for all women since women constitute half the world. The issue of representativeness (or unrepresentativeness) in fact crops up in all social movement and user group debates and is often used as an excuse for not taking users seriously. Service users and their organisations can expect to be criticised as unrepresentative. This will tend to happen particularly when service providers, local authorities and others do not like what users have to say and regard it as a threat to the status quo and to their own power and influence, or when they are so unused to hearing users speak out that they assume anyone who has learnt to do so cannot be 'typical' (Beresford and Campbell, 1994). Beresford and Campbell (1994), in a closely argued paper, suggest that it is up to the service world itself to ensure representative involvement. This can be done, they propose, by adopting less tokenistic forms of involvement than inviting just one or two people to speak on behalf of many, by providing appropriate forms of access and support, by involving a diversity of users (including those from black and minority ethnic communities) and by inviting members of collective advocacy organisations to speak for the organisation, not just for themselves. Professionals should also recognise, say these authors, that they themselves have not established their representativeness and that, however narrow the base of those speaking out, this can never excuse bad practice. Furthermore, whereas the current fashion for focus groups, market research and other centrally controlled forms of consultation does not involve any element of power-sharing with service users, conversely, user groups and movements do organise collectively, mandate their representatives to speak on their behalf, and often represent views and perspectives gathered through the widest possible participation. The authors conclude with a challenge that resonates loudly with the research reported in this book:

> There are important questions here for service agencies. Can they reconcile schemes for user involvement and empowerment within the overall political structures within which they are set? How can such schemes avoid being marginal and tokenistic?
>
> (ibid.: 324)

Later chapters will attempt to provide some answers from the experience of abused women.

Loss of integrity or loss of impetus

Even alternatives to mainstream statutory and voluntary services that are user-controlled from the start can face problems. They may adopt what Dowson (1997) calls 'the service culture' of managerial and evaluative structures, and may become complicit with the statutory services. Alternatively, they may start to mimic traditional services over time, rather than breaking new ground to meet actual needs in more appropriate ways (O'Hagan, 1993), the biggest challenge in doing something different being 'to keep it different' (Lindow, 1994: 9). Lindow suggests that ways of doing this include: constantly raising the awareness of new members, keeping power in the hands of users, remaining true to the group's original philosophy and avoiding the replication of traditional, hierarchical management structures and undemocratic leadership.

Power: how it operates

If empowerment is about sharing or taking power, as we have suggested earlier, then it becomes important to think in both theoretical and practical ways about what that power is and how it operates. Some ways of looking at power hold out more hope than others for service users. For example, postmodernist views of 'bottom-up' power and resistance can be helpful, although the challenge they imply to the grand theories that can inspire collective action has been something of a dampener.

Power, though a fundamental aspect of people's lives and something we can all talk about in a common-sense way, is actually one of the most disputed and contested of all concepts (Scott, 1994). In our attempts to understand and explain how power operates within society, difficulties begin when we try to formulate precise definitions. No definition of power has universal support among sociologists and political scientists, because what we think power is, and how and why it is possessed and exercised, depends on disciplinary conventions, theoretical perspectives and political allegiances. Emancipatory theories tend to involve a call for power, and our understanding of it, to be transformed, so that power can be shared in new ways for the good of the wider society (Mullender and Ward, 1991; Dullea and Mullender, 1999). We need to look in more detail at what is meant by this.

Power as domination

Many analyses of power (e.g. Croft and Beresford, 1996; Servian, 1996) start with the work of Lukes, an Oxford sociologist and political scientist. Lukes's definition is that 'A exercises power over B when A affects B in a manner contrary to B's interests' (1974: 34). His three-dimensional view of power builds up in three distinct stages. First, in the one-dimensional view, decisions are made as a result of 'actual, observable conflict' (ibid.: 13). There is no allowance for interests that might be 'unarticulated or unobservable' (ibid.: 13). Rather, they are consciously held preferences that result in actions related to overt issues. Out-and-out sexism versus consciously aware feminism would fall under this definition. However, women know only too well that most opposition is more subtle than this, and that it is often harder to marshall the arguments against unspoken patriarchal assumptions that men know best and are always in the right.

Lukes's two-dimensional view is about keeping certain issues off the agenda. Overt, observable conflict is not the whole story. The sheer power of the patriarchy, we might argue, has been in making it so difficult for women, for centuries, even to question the way they were treated and expected to live their lives. There was simply no debate, no issue. Any woman who did attempt to speak out was vilified and rejected, often by other women who wanted to keep their reputations in the eyes of society, quite as much as by men. Lukes traces various ideas of coercion and more subtle influence operating as barriers to the open debate of policy issues that it would not suit one interested party to have brought into the open. 'Non-decisions' (ibid.: 18) become as important as decisions, with demonstrable vested interests built into the prevailing political process and an uphill battle for anyone who happens to think the whole system, and its underpinning value base, is wrong. This is certainly what it has felt like, over the years, when women have tried to question their lot. Men's interests have seemed to be embedded in the entire political, judicial and religious system. One of us can remember laughing out loud, for example, at the incongruity of a radio station inviting the chief commentators in a public debate, over a lesbian woman wanting a hospital to help her have a baby by artificial insemination, to be a senior churchman, a judge and a doctor (all male). How would the deeper questions about women's sexuality and motherhood ever enter into consideration on the same terms as these men's learned pronouncements, backed as they were by all the weight of traditional authority – that is, of power? And the same thing is true of woman abuse, perhaps most starkly in child contact cases where women opposing contact with abusive ex-partners have been accused in court of 'implacable hostility' or of generating 'parental alienation syndrome' because no one would listen to their deepest fears that they and their children were still in danger (Radford *et al.*, 1999; Saunders, 2001). So, as well as fostering certain decisions, power is used to shape people's perceptions, cognitions and preferences so that they accept their role in the existing order of things, because they see this as either natural and unchangeable, or divinely ordained and beneficial, or inevitable because no kind of change is likely to be possible. All these suggestions have been used to keep women 'in their place'.

Lukes adds a third dimension to his model by arguing that the study of power cannot be confined to conflict that is observable in the way those with opposing interests behave, even if we include the way issues are kept off the agenda. That is still an inadequate view of the world, he continues, because power is used, not only to suppress conflict, but also to stop it arising in the first place. At this most subtle level, the status quo is so pervasive (1974: 21) that the system reinforces itself without conscious choice or even the conscious exercise of power. No action is necessary; there are no acts of conflict. The less powerful party does what the powerful party wants him or her to do, but feels as if they have chosen it for themselves. Their very 'thoughts and desires' (ibid.: 23) have been controlled. This is how advertising works and it will also sound very familiar to anyone who has lived with an abusive man. It is 'thought control' and 'indoctrination' (ibid.: 23), but at a very insidious, subtle and completely legal level that depends on the utter belief of the person or group with the power that that power is absolute, right, legitimate and unquestionable. Again, think of abusive men, and of the role of law, church and state in upholding their position over the centuries. For empowerment to happen, not only must resources be acquired to influence the outcomes of overt decisions, and access be secured to decision-making processes, but, also, political consciousness must be raised, so that women, service users and other historically powerless groups begin to perceive the issues that affect their lives and the need to become involved in these. This begins to feel much closer to the way in which feminist activists view the world and was certainly how the women's movement came to establish the first refuges.

Power: relational

A fourth dimension to the study of power has been added by the French philosopher, Michel Foucault, in an enormously influential analysis that might better be seen perhaps as a departure from all previous notions. For Foucault, power is not a possession, to be won and lost in struggles between different classes and social groupings or between them and the state (Foucault, 1979). Power, in this unitary sense, in his view, does not exist 'out there' as a separate entity. We can no longer talk about 'social structural oppression' in the way we formerly did when discussing the patriarchal subordination of women. Power is often seen rather, in these post-structuralist days, as 'an effect of the operation of social relationships, between groups and between individuals', so that '[e]very group and every individual exercises power and is subjected to it' (Sheridan, 1980: 218). This happens at every interaction and at every moment within any inter-action, in constantly unequal and shifting ways. In other words, power is everywhere, contained within every kind of interpersonal or social relation-ship and transaction, whether economic, informational, discursive, sexual or of any other kind, and even people whose ability to exercise power in most directions is severely curtailed generally find some other outlet (Sheridan, 1980). Poor black men experiencing racism at work and on the streets, who at home are woman abusers, might be seen as one example of this, though this in no way excuses their abuse nor places it outside their control to end it (see Williams, 2003).

Furthermore, in Foucault's (1979) world-view, wherever there is power, there is resistance, contained within the same interaction. This leads to the conclusion that everyone has some ability to resist his or her own oppres-sion or abuse – to exercise 'bottom-up' power. We nowadays see that women experiencing violence typically explore a whole range of survival mechanisms and do 'fight back' against their abusers in any way they can (Okun, 1986; Hoff, 1990; Kirkwood, 1993). However, it is rare for the 'plurality of resistances, each a special case, distributed in an irregular way in time and space' to converge 'to bring about a major upheaval' because 'resistance [like power] usually takes the form of innumerable, mobile, transitory points' (Sheridan, 1980: 185). In other words, resistance is every-where, but everywhere it resides in individuals and is continually shifting, not constant or shared in a form that can be got hold of and worked with. Revolution *is* possible, but, according to Foucault, would depend on the 'strategic codification' of all these points of resistance into a concerted effort, in the same way as the state draws together and institutes the dynamics of power (Foucault, 1979: 96). The women's movement, des-cribed in the last chapter, can therefore be seen as an extraordinary achieve-ment, while the potential for holding on to and further advancing its gains is the responsibility of each one of us, in every daily interaction, and arguably might not normally have an influence beyond that particular interaction.

Foucault's notion of power is a useful corrective to approaches which, in trying to overcome women's position as discriminated against, actually replicate and perpetuate discourses that position the female as victim within a fixed identity. On the other hand, it could be argued that Foucault's formulation of power makes it impossible to analyse – and even rejects the existence of – patriarchy; that is, the systematic power of men as a group over women as a group. This makes it much harder for feminism to survive or to be helpful as a body of theory because it can be accused of being essentialist, of being a unitary and overarching 'grand theory' that is now too simplistic to be taken seriously. As we indicated in the last chapter, much feminist scholarship has gone into contesting and debating these charges, leading to substantial development within feminist epistemology (see, for example, Hill Collins, 1991; Stacey, 1993; Stanley and Wise, 1993) and to a recent tendency to refer to 'feminisms' rather than 'feminism' (see Squires and Kemp, 1997).

Certainly, we can no longer assume, just because a project or initiative is set up to serve women, that it is automatically good for all women. It takes work to ensure inclusivity in relation to ethnicity, sexuality, socio-economic status, (dis)ability and age, for example, to engage creatively with difference and to combat discrimination. When establishing or evaluating any service, it is important to ask: 'which women benefit, how much, at what costs, compared to which alternatives' (Rhode, 1989: 317). At the same time, there is a need to avoid excessive fragmentation. Practice cannot be based on an individualism that denies common experiences of abuse and violence, any more than essentialist assumptions of universal justice must be allowed to deny individual difference or diversity. There is still the potential for an 'emancipatory project' in social welfare (Leonard, 1997), and theorists in Australia (Pease and Fook, 1999; Healy, 2000) and the UK (Batsleer and Humphries, 2000) have extended this thinking into detailed possibilities for 'critical', 'progressive' or 'transformative' practice.

The critique of 'grand theories', or meta-narratives, as progressivist and positivist has been a threat to feminism in some ways (see, for example, Harding, 1993, writing within the feminist standpoint tradition). Feminism has had to adapt to encompass the fragmented and multiple subjectivities that we now consider to constitute 'woman'. However, since feminism is a body of theory that is actually very good at handling uncertainty, relativism, dissent and questioning of the discourses through which people make sense of their lives and their world, it is still viable to think about women as women, and about the multiple oppressions that different groups of women sustain, provided we can encompass difference and diversity within this.

Following on from many structuralist, socialist and standpoint approaches, postmodernism and post-structuralism have particularly emphasised that knowledge is historically and culturally specific and that we must listen to the voices of individuals previously silenced by dominant discourses if we are to understand and work with them, for example through helping them tell their own stories in ways that explore relations of power and control. Foucault's analysis of power makes it particularly important to hear individual voices and individual narratives in both practice and research (Davis, 1994). There is not one 'true' or 'authentic' voice (Edwards and Ribbens, 1998). Rather, we need to hear many women – including women from black and minority ethnic communities, disabled, lesbian and older women and women living in poverty – all talking about their personal lives and their experiences in family, community and society. We then have a responsibility to attempt to convey publicly the understandings and experiences they share, without losing meaning or context (Ribbens, 1998). Certainly, it has been our aim throughout the study reported here, and now in this book, to raise the voices of women who have experienced abuse and who have sought help from various sources thereafter.

Of particular relevance in this context, perhaps, Foucauldian views on power, as outlined above, lead us to infer that there is power inherent in the responses made by professionals to abuse and that individual women receiving services may resist the superiority or subordination implied in the relationship between helper and helped. Hearing women's voices in respect of policy and practice is just as important as hearing them in relation to the original abuse. Failure to do so can lead to equally inappropriate responses in both cases. Personal experience, pain and suffering *can* form an underpinning for collective action through 'the valid therapeutic contribution of the non-expert, and the centrality of personal experience as a powerful tool for change' (Campbell, 1996: 221). All user movements can bring together the personal and the political – for example, impairment at the level of personal feelings, emotions, perceptions and pain, with disability at the level of social structural relations (Morris, 1996; Beresford, 1997) – just as the women's movement does. These are the messages with which we shall conclude this chapter. Listening to and working in partnership with abused women is not optional. It has to be the way forward for multi-agency and other domestic violence services.

Conclusion

Much of the literature and research reviewed above on user participation as a route to changing the distribution of power in organisations appears pessimistic. The contemporary analysis of power that sees it as everywhere and nowhere – far harder to get hold of and to oppose than we historically thought – is apparently of little help in this process, except that it does show how every individual can and does resist, at every point and all the time. However, we have to find a way forward, one that takes into account all the obstacles and complexities we have reviewed in this chapter. Not to do so will leave service users, including abused women, without a voice, excluded from decision-making and without a real say in their own lives (Croft and Beresford, 1996). So, rather than continuing with 'outside in' social policy and sociological commentary in the rest of this book, we will move to an approach that aims to get inside and to find out what can perhaps work better. A key theme is the need to be willing to develop ideas and responses that enable women survivors to engage with what exists in terms of services and forums, to work out what gains can be made in any given situation, and to develop a more sophisticated understanding of the operation of power. Within this, it is important not to lose sight of the fact that refuges and related provision are among the very few feminist organisations that have been established in the UK (McIntosh, 1996). These achievements did not come easily and they certainly cannot be sustained or improved through tokenistic rhetoric. They have been the hallmark of women's resistance and campaigning, and their survival is testimony to the fact that they are still needed in contemporary life.

Despite the difficulties, user involvement is crucial in improving agency responses to domestic abuse. This is all the more true since '[e]ffective action in any social sphere is impossible without an adequate understanding of the nature and extent of the problem' (Mullender, 1996: 1), yet violence against women remains surrounded by widespread ignorance. We need to draw on the expertise of women service users as citizens, as social actors, as no longer socially excluded. If they are to share control over the design and delivery of services, this means having a real voice in refuges, domestic violence forums, key statutory agencies and other groups. Women's power to resist oppression includes the oppression that can come from services themselves, for example services that started life with feminist principles but may have allowed them to be diluted along the way. Of course, there is difference and diversity between women, and services must be responsive accordingly. The range of voices we shall hear in the chapters that follow will help to ensure that this is the case.

Part 2

Women's views and voices in domestic violence services

Chapter 4

What abused women think of the services they receive

In the previous chapters in Part 1, we developed arguments about the frequent exclusion of women and of gender issues from theorising on service user movements, and about the contributions these movements make, together with the barriers they face in becoming effective. We also discussed the way in which women who have experienced violence are rarely seen as forming a service user group in their own right and so miss out on the possible benefits and strengths which could result.

In the following chapters, we build on these debates to put forward arguments about the frequent exclusion of abused women in practical terms from decision-making within domestic violence policy and about concrete ways of challenging and improving the current situation. Many of the sensitive issues, contradictions and complexities which have been drawn out theoretically in the preceding section will be developed in the ensuing chapters in practical ways and in specific relation to current domestic violence policy and practice in the UK. In this section (Part 2) of the book, we will discuss what women survivors of violence think of the services they receive and how much their voices are heard. We will also look at why the involvement of domestic violence service users is essential to the policy process. The final section (Part 3) contains chapters on how to go about it, on the practical difficulties and positives involved and on examples of good and innovatory practice in regard to service user participation and accountability to abuse survivors.

Throughout, we will draw extensively on the findings and insights of the study on raising abused women's voices to which we referred in the Introduction, and which was one of the studies within the recent Economic and Social Research Council's Violence Research Programme (see Hague *et al.*, 2001, 2002). Conducted by the present authors, it examined how much the voices of abused women are heard in service and policy development. This chapter also draws on the Briefing Notes for the Home Office (prepared by two of the present authors) on women survivors of abuse and their views of the services they have received (Mullender and Hague, 2000), and on the wider review of these issues on which the Home Office

Briefing Notes were based (later published as Mullender and Hague, 2001). Many personal testimonies and accounts have been produced by domestic violence survivors themselves, accompanied by the publication of numerous self-help books and academic accounts of women's help-seeking efforts (e.g. Homer *et al.*, 1984; Women's Aid, 1989; Hoff, 1990; Kirkwood, 1993; *Violence Against Lesbians in the Home*, 1998), and we have also drawn on these. In the present chapter, we will begin by considering how, under the impetus of the women's activist movement, domestic violence provision has been transformed, compared to how it was in the past. We will then go on to discuss the views of abused women service users, from the 1980s onwards, of the services they have received, followed by a consideration, first of diversity and equality issues, then of the performance of individual agencies as far as survivors of abuse are concerned. The chapter concludes by bringing the debate right up to date and considering very recent research and the current situation.

Thus, we begin these discussions by again, as in the previous chapters, affirming that any consideration of the views of domestic violence survivors needs to start by acknowledging the social movement that has been listening and responding to the needs of abused women for the last thirty years. Throughout, the empowerment of women has been the watchword of this activist movement of women, as discussed throughout this book. Its principles include both an adherence to an analysis of domestic violence based on understandings of gender and power, and also a stated commitment to raising the voices of abused women and children and to insisting that society, men, the state and both statutory and voluntary sector agencies take the abuse of women seriously (see Dobash and Dobash, 1992; Mullender and Hague, 2001). Developing out of the wider women's movement, understandings of men's violence towards women that are derived directly, and in a principled way, from women's actual experiences have, since the 1970s, informed both feminist theories and practice (see, for example, Schechter, 1982; Kelly, 1988; Dobash and Dobash, 1992; Hague and Malos, 1998). Over the years, feminist-inspired projects and campaigns have grown out of, and attempted to respond to, these direct experiences.

Indeed, as we have discussed in Chapter 2, the very first responses to domestic violence in the mid 1970s came about through the self-organisation of women's groups and women's centres connected with the Women's Liberation Movement of the time. Safe houses and refuges were established by women for women, with a strong element of self-help and collective activity by survivors themselves (Dobash and Dobash, 1992; Hague and Malos, 1998). Since then, emergency and long-term housing, advocacy and outreach projects, helplines and women's support groups have continued to be established by women's organisations (which often themselves contain a high percentage of domestic violence survivors), despite a persistent lack of stable funding. Thus, over the years, women who have had personal experience of domestic violence have played a key role in instigating such services, helping to ensure that these have been sensitive to abused women's expressed needs and wishes, as part of the wider movement.

The activist movement against domestic violence in the UK includes campaigning and lobbying bodies, autonomous refuge and support organisations, a wide variety of women's groups and the four Women's Aid national federations, as we have outlined previously. While independent refuge groups do exist, the federations co-ordinate the majority of the provision of refuge services, alongside a network of refuges for women from minority communities, including a variety of Asian women's projects. Women's Aid lobbies and campaigns on domestic violence, with the federations acting as the principal specialist organisations across the UK offering protection to abused women and their children and representing their views and interests. The refuge movement has always had strong principles and policies concerned in direct practical ways with making sure that abused women and children are listened to and recognised. Other grass-roots women's projects and campaigning groups have also consistently voiced both the injustices experienced by abused women and their children and also their visions for the future, their hopes and their needs (Women's Aid Federation of England, 1998; Southall Black Sisters, 2000). Imkaan, for example, assists the network of Asian women's refuges, facilitating network-building and providing training, conferences and research, geared towards the stated needs of Asian women in the UK. Southall Black Sisters has, for many years, campaigned on violence against women, and particularly takes up issues which affect immigrant women and women from minority ethnic communities, informed by the words and views of the women themselves. Many of these organisations have been campaigning and listening to women's voices and needs since long before the subject of domestic violence began tentatively to move into the mainstream.

Now, though, mainstreaming is with us. After years – indeed millennia – of neglect, domestic violence by men against women is in the public view as never before. The abuse of women in intimate and family situations has become a major issue of concern within social policy, social work, child protection and public education, and among many members of the public in the UK, as elsewhere in countries across the globe. The result has been the development of new services, good practice and policy guidance, improved initiatives within the police, and the setting up of inter-agency domestic violence forums. These previously unprecedented responses to domestic abuse are as yet, uneven and are often not prioritised within complex budgetary demands and competing interests faced by local authorities, the health service and the criminal justice system. But they are there.

The increase in service provision, though dogged by scarce resources, has been welcomed by long-term practitioners and activists in the field and by survivors of domestic violence – sometimes with a certain measure of disbelief (see Hague and Malos, 1998; Taylor-Browne, 2001).

It is quite clear, although it is sometimes overlooked by present-day policy-makers, that much of this new attention has its roots in the movement against domestic violence and that – without this movement – the subsequent improvements and changes would not have happened (Dobash and Dobash, 1992; Harwin, 1999). Thus, over the years, activism, backed up by research and service development, has transformed both our understandings of the issue and the practice of many agencies throughout the statutory and voluntary sectors, as we indicated in Chapter 2. But we might ask whether what survivors of domestic violence think and feel, their views and their aspirations, have been taken on as an integral part of this transformation or merely whether professionals have been taking over. In Part 1, we looked at this question in a theoretical way. Here, we look at it more practically. How do abused women view the services, which have been offered to them, and do these services meet their needs and enable them to increase their personal safety and to build violence-free futures for themselves and their children?

Domestic violence survivors and inadequate services

It is almost impossible now to remember the old days when no services whatsoever were available in the UK. The domestic violence field has changed beyond all recognition since the early 1970s. (For a consideration of how domestic violence was viewed between 1945 and 1970, see Hague and Wilson, 1996, 2000.) However, in more recent years, despite the transformations which we have highlighted, women's experiences of all the public sector services have consistently been that they are patchy and inadequate, with practitioners often assuming judgmental or woman-blaming attitudes. This was the case especially up until the mid 1990s. For example, two key studies in the 1980s illuminated women's help-seeking efforts at the time and the difficulties and barriers which they faced at every turn (Binney et al., 1981; Dobash et al., 1985). Many women in these and subsequent studies have spoken of trying one agency after another and of the long trek between them to find help, sometimes leading to an ever increasing sense of desperation and disillusion.

The previous lack of attention accorded to violence experienced by women and, indeed, the fact that it has been sanctioned throughout history (Dobash and Dobash, 1980; Pleck, 1986), have continued to have their effects, despite service improvements. In the 1980s, there were various attempts to work with women in respectful ways and to recognise them as active participants in trying to stop the violence they had experienced. Nevertheless, women survivors of violence have continued to be stereo-typed, very often, in public discourse and among helping agencies as passive and incapable (Aris *et al.*, 2002). Despite the efforts of the Women's Aid movement, abused women are still rarely regarded as com-petent participants in the policy process. Their views of the inadequacy of services have, until recently, fallen on deaf ears, despite document after document detailing these difficulties (Smith, 1989; Women's Aid, 1989; Hague *et al.*, 1996a).

As regards individual agencies, there have been clear improvements in service provision and delivery in the last ten years. Nevertheless, it continues to be well researched that all of the public sector organisations tend to suffer from internal inconsistency and that responses also vary substantially between different geographical localities (Malos and Hague, 1993; Grace, 1995; Taylor-Browne, 2001). Abused women talk of feeling constantly let down and of unsatisfactory responses, despite attempts by agencies to improve (Humphreys *et al.*, 2000). While positive assessments by women of services received are becoming more common, many women users have continued to end up with very negative views of the whole range of agencies involved in their and their children's lives.

Government is currently trying to catch up. In 1999, the Women's Unit of the Cabinet Office (now named the Women and Equality Unit and moved to the Department of Trade and Industry) published an action plan for violence against women (Cabinet Office, 1999). This action plan was far from comprehensive, but was a beginning nonetheless. It was accompanied in 2000 by the production by the Home Office of a useful set of Briefing Notes summarising what works in tackling domestic violence. These devel-opments, among other official initiatives, were important in terms of signalling a new willingness by government to take on the issue. The Briefing Notes detailed both inadequacies in services and also innovative new developments within different agencies and policy agendas (Home Office, 2000). They provided evidence that, currently, many committed attempts are being made across the field to improve the way that agencies deal with domestic violence. Indeed, the Home Office Crime Reduction Programme on Violence Against Women, established after the Briefing Notes were produced, has since funded a varied set of demonstration projects to give some pointers for co-ordinated ways forward in the future. In some of these projects, concerted efforts to find out abused women's views have been conducted and satisfaction with services received has increased in consequence. The Cheshire Domestic Violence Outreach Service, for instance, has conducted and published qualitative surveys of what service users think of the service and the project team has acted on the results (Cheshire Domestic Abuse Project, 2002). More commonly, though, it seems that women, as yet, remain dissatisfied and unsafe even after they have sought help in a systematic manner and made use of all the relevant services that are available.

It is not only women who urgently need improved services. We now know that domestic violence can have varied and serious impacts on children who witness, live with or otherwise experience it (see Mullender and Morley, 1994; Hester *et al.*, 2000). However, outside refuges (Hague *et al.*, 1996a), children's voices are very rarely heard in relation to their views about the abuse experienced by adults and about policy and practice responses. Until recently, for example, studies of domestic violence and children in the UK used mothers and professionals as their research respondents, although recent work (McGee, 2000; Mullender *et al.*, 2002) includes consultation with children. A study in the Economic and Social Research Council's Children 5–16 years: Growing into the 21st Century Research Programme (Mullender *et al.*, 2002) has revealed that children are far from being passive victims of domestic violence. Rather, they use a wide range of coping strategies, often in an active way, to deal with the violence they experience. The research found that children would, generally speaking, like to be consulted about responses, and that they can be a rich source of good advice for other children and adults (see also Mullender *et al.*, 2000). However, while there are many new practice developments within agencies in regard to domestic violence that attempt to address children's needs, once again few of these have consulted children directly. Relevant agencies could usefully seek the views of children who have experience of domestic violence (in a sensitive and careful way and where it is safe to do so) about policy and services. Scottish Women's Aid, for example, published *Young People Say* in 1998 (Scottish Women's Aid, 1998). Many Women's Aid refuges run children's workshops and hold regular, decision-making children's meetings, but few other agencies do anything comparable.

Diversity and services

The situation of potential exclusion and silencing for both abused women and their children is often compounded for minority groups. Black women and children may experience institutional and personal racism, for example, and often face added problems when attempting to access services, as well as those experienced by all women, as detailed in research by Amina Mama (Mama, 1996). In her pioneering survey of statutory and voluntary sector responses, conducted in the 1980s, the women interviewed had consistently encountered unsatisfactory and discriminatory services, as well as overtly racist attitudes. Activist and first-hand accounts such as those published by Southall Black Sisters (1990) have confirmed these concerns. A study in the 1990s in the London borough of Islington (James-Hanman, 1995) suggested that provision still failed to meet language and cultural needs, leaving many black and minority ethnic women isolated, unaware of their options and sometimes placed in additional danger by discriminatory responses by helping agencies. More recently, Rai and Thiara (1997, 1999) have provided two helpful overviews of refuge and other support services from the perspective of black service users and workers. Black organisations in the community are valued according to their studies, but other sources of help are commonly perceived by women as not understanding the black experience and sometimes as institutionally racist, particularly (although, by no means, solely) in predominantly white areas. A new study, named *Domestic Violence and Minoritisation: Supporting women to independence*, similarly describes discriminatory responses continuing in a range of agencies including some refuges (Batsleer *et al.*, 2002).

For lesbian and bisexual women and their children, domestic violence from past or recent male partners, or from women partners, can present particular difficulties which are often compounded by homophobia (*Violence Against Lesbians in the Home*, 1998). These may include negative, prejudiced or voyeuristic attitudes within agencies and lack of information about the issue, leading to inappropriate or judgmental responses. Lesbians are often even more silenced in relation to violence issues than other women, and stand even less chance than others of being recognised by, and acknowledged within, the policy process.

Disabled women and children are also likely to experience additional difficulties, which may be exacerbated by negative attitudes and discrimination. For example, a disabled woman living in her own home faces the potential of being trapped there, and may be unable to access services or publicity about them (James-Hanman, 1994). It is difficult for a disabled woman to leave home if she is not mobile or if she has had her home adapted. Further, a complex care package may also have been assembled to support her which may be hard to leave behind (Cross, 1999). All of these situations are likely to be seriously exacerbated if her abuser is also her carer. Leaving situations of abuse may be almost impossible if accessible refuge accommodation is over-subscribed, which it often is. Deaf women face particular problems where no interpreting in sign language is available and where agencies are unaware and ignorant of, or insensitive to, deaf issues. The list goes on and on (Mullender and Hague, 2001). However, disabled women's views on these complex difficulties relating to domestic violence are rarely heard, if ever, even within disability movement organisations. Overall, the voices of abused women and children from minority groups of all types are inadequately represented in the literature and in policy documentation, with resulting implications for potentially skewed and discriminatory policy development.

It should not be thought, of course, that agencies do not try to deal with these issues. Some do, although not always with a great deal of success, often due to resource shortfalls (for example, in refuges). A few have begun to be more sensitive and inclusive about equality matters overall and about consultation in general. For example, some specialist police units (e.g. community safety units in London) that deal with racial, homophobic and domestic violence have begun to develop increased awareness about issues for disabled, black and lesbian women. Policies and good practice guidelines on domestic abuse within a variety of agencies may stipulate listening to what abused women have to say, and new service plans or reviews conducted by partnerships and local authorities may include some consultation on user satisfaction with the relevant services, including specialist provision for minority groups.

Individual agencies

Individual agencies vary in their responsiveness to domestic violence, so that it is worth discussing women's views of each in turn. Starting with those agencies which have a connection to the activist movement, women's organisations and refuge groups provide a wide range of emergency refuge, support, outreach and advocacy services, which have a generally good record of involving service users in both provision and policy. Abused women, including those from minority groups, consistently rate refuge and outreach services very positively within both personal testimonies and research surveys. For example, in study after study, refuges have elicited by far the most satisfaction from women who have used them, as compared with other agencies (Malos and Hague, 1993; Hague *et al.*, 1996; Humphreys *et al.*, 2000; Mullender and Hague, 2001). In the majority of cases, refuge organisations are the principal agencies that offer supportive and understanding staff, expert in dealing with domestic violence, and they are frequently the only ones that women believe can offer them safety. Conversely, mainstream agencies often pay too little attention to safety, according, for example, to over half the women surveyed through a self-completion questionnaire widely circulated in Lewisham (London Borough of Lewisham Community Safety Team, 1998). It is also the case that refuge staff are generally the only professionals to whom abused women feel able to tell the full details of their experiences because, in most other contexts, they may fear disbelief, patronising responses, blame and possible consequences in terms of child protection intervention (Sissons, 1999; Kelly and Humphreys, 2001; Mullender and Hague, 2001).

While there are always, of course, improvements that could be made, and the crowded conditions of many refuges continue to be rated negatively by users of the service, the generally positive tone of the feedback on refuge provision is more or less universal. For example, Henderson (1997) found that 81 per cent of women surveyed in Scotland had found Women's Aid services to be helpful, owing to both the actual assistance provided and the supportive attitudes of staff. Women's support groups and advice or information services are also valued highly. An independent evaluation of support groups for women survivors of domestic violence in the US found that women attending them experienced substantial improvements in social and emotional functioning and also a reduction in violence (Tutty *et al.*, 1993).

Specialist projects for women and children from minority communities have a key part to play. As we have noted previously, the network of Asian women's refuges and support groups in towns and cities across the UK operates both within and alongside Women's Aid, offering culturally appropriate and non-racist support. In some localities, there are also a few specialist refuge organisations and support groups variously, for example, for all black women and children, or for African, for African Caribbean, for Chinese, for Jewish and for other women and children from minority ethnic communities. Mama's study (1996) found some dissatisfaction among black women escaping violence with generalist refuges, as compared with specialist ones. However, the Women's Aid federations have attempted to address some of these problems with specific work on refuges and black women (see e.g. Rai and Thiara, 1997) and through the adoption of strategies to combat racism and other forms of discrimination. These strategies are not as yet completely effective, and a recent study has noted continued difficulties for black and minority ethnic women in generalist refuges in some areas (Batsleer *et al.*, 2002). However, in general terms, Rai and Thiara report that black women value refuges highly. There are also a very few specialist refuges of other types, for example, for women with learning disabilities, for women who have experienced sexual assault and for young women, all of which are generally rated highly by service users. Similarly, *Violence Against Lesbians in the Home*, while encouraging further improvements, states of refuges: 'it is unlikely that any agency has responded more positively to Lesbians fleeing violence in the home' (1998: 50).

As regards other agencies, the police are a vital emergency service for victims of domestic violence, and have a central role in meeting the needs of abused women and their children. They frequently top the list of agencies contacted for help, and the major improvements in policing policy which we have witnessed over the last decade have been broadly supported by women who have experienced domestic violence and by their advocacy organisations, such as Women's Aid (Home Office, 1990, 2000a). Even so, in some localities, women continue to report little change in police and criminal justice responses with only patchy improvements recorded across the country as a whole (though these are undoubtedly considerable in some areas and are continuing to get better) (Grace, 1995; Plotnikoff and Woolfson, 1998; Home Office, 2000).

A 1999 study by Liz Kelly and colleagues in London, supported by Henderson's (1997) research in Scotland and related work nationwide, found that domestic violence survivors are often quite clear about the services they need from the police. In the Kelly study, for example, women said that they wanted respectful treatment by, and assertive action from, the police, but that they did not always receive either or both. They thought that domestic violence should be responded to as a crime, but they needed support and protection in order for this to be a viable option as far as their own participation as witnesses was concerned. There were major problems in translating arrest into effective action against perpetrators and, where prosecutions did occur, the sentences passed were perceived by victims as failing to place sanctions on men's behaviour (Kelly, 1999).

Like the police, social services have a vital role to play, both through their adult and their children's services. Most studies have found that, despite the difficulties to which we alluded in Chapter 3, women value the practical help available from social workers (Binney et al., 1981; Pahl, 1985; Mullender, 1996; Humphreys and Mullender, 2002). They commonly approach social services for help and advice, despite the fear reported in most of the relevant studies (e.g. Abrahams, 1994; Mullender et al., 2002) that they might lose their children through child protection procedures. However, there is little evidence of abused women being able to influence social services' responses, despite some increase in awareness in recent years (Humphreys et al., 2000).

Similarly, in the NHS and the health field, services have improved considerably, but not nearly enough. Health practitioners have a key role to play in meeting abused women's needs, both in terms of physical injuries and of mental health problems such as anxiety, depression and insomnia (Mooney, 1994; Williamson, 2000). Thus, it is vital that health services are able to respond effectively, quickly and sympathetically to women experiencing domestic violence, but there is much evidence that health personnel often do not ask about the violence, or that women in the situation may feel too anxious to disclose it (Williamson, 2000). In one recent study, for example, the unsympathetic manner of some practitioners and their evident lack of time constituted further obstacles for women, who were not satisfied with being prescribed antidepressants or sleeping tablets (e.g. Dominy and Radford, 1996). However, specific, practical improvements in health responses and the adoption of a more proactive approach are now taking place with the development of a variety of initiatives. These include the adoption of practice guidelines by the Royal Colleges and the specialist practitioner organisations for groups of health workers, and the publication of a Department of Health resource manual (Department of Health, 2000).

According to survivors' testimonies and to research evidence, one of the principal needs of women and children escaping violence in the home is for access to safe and secure temporary and permanent housing options – in other words, for somewhere safe to go. While temporary housing may be provided by the refuge movement, or through the homelessness legislation, access to permanent housing is a more problematic issue. Women and children who are statutorily homeless due to domestic violence under the homelessness legislation make extensive use of local authority and housing association provision, and their treatment by their local housing department is of key importance in this respect. Women survivors consistently make the same points during housing consultation exercises and wider-scale research projects with housing-related content (e.g. Malos and Hague, 1993; Henderson, 1997; Morley, 2000). In summary, they regularly highlight the need for a sympathetic, believing approach, a non-judgmental service, an ending of unreasonable delays in being accepted as homeless and in being rehoused and the removal of obstacles to service (e.g. the requirement for certain forms of proof or the insistence that legal remedies to remove the perpetrator be substituted for rehousing the woman and children). Interviewees in all of these studies consistently stressed that the safety of abused women and their children should be the major priority, with a strong emphasis on confidentiality and security, and on the need for both emergency and permanent housing to be available, secure and of a reasonable standard in an area the survivor considers safe.

While there are many other individual agencies to which abused women turn for help, there is particular potential when dealing with domestic violence (which crosses so many areas of work and cannot be corralled into just one category) for improved service co-ordination and integration. This is usually carried out through inter-agency initiatives, as encouraged by both the present and the previous governments (Home Office, 1995, 1999; Hague, 2000). The only national study to date in the UK of multi-agency initiatives as a response to domestic violence (see Hague et al., 1996; Hague, 2000, 2001) found that domestic violence forums and other inter-agency responses could sometimes take a creative approach to tackling domestic violence, but that they could also become 'talking shop' exercises, as noted previously, and that women experiencing violence were rarely involved. In this study, some of the ideas which women survivors themselves suggested to the research team (by no means a comprehensive list) included:

- listening to women;
- questionnaires on the effectiveness of forums and services;
- snappy slogans and campaigns;
- more publicity and public awareness campaigns;
- more involvement of abused women in worker training sessions and in domestic violence training overall;
- more participation of abused women in new services established by forums;
- the setting up of a local domestic violence ombudsperson post in the community;

- a principled avoiding of the exploitation or 'using' of women participants;
- adequate compensation for time spent on consultation and other forms of participation, plus expenses;
- using refuges to pass information between survivors and multi-agency initiatives.

(Hague *et al.*, 1996)

Across the board, however, it seems that, despite focused suggestions of this type from women survivors, they are rarely actioned. More commonly, documents in which abused women's voices are raised continue to describe inefficient or self-serving policies, cutbacks and a lack of helpful resources in the right places at the right time (Mama, 1996; Hague and Malos, 1998; Mullender and Hague, 2001). In sum, then, women's experiences of services and agencies over the years have commonly been that they are under-resourced, difficult to access and of uncertain effectiveness (e.g. Dobash *et al.*, 1985; Mullender, 1996; Home Office, 2000), and that these difficulties may be compounded for minority groups by discrimination and disadvantage (James-Hanman, 1994; Mama, 1996; Rai and Thiara, 1997). Things have of course improved since the mid to late 1990s with very significant and positive changes in recent years. Professionals in the field can take some solace from the widespread development of new policy and practice. Unfortunately, though, women and children escaping abuse still face inadequate services in many instances and change remains localised and incomplete.

The current situation

Bringing the debate right up to the moment, wide-ranging consultation is being carried out by government in 2003 on the proposed new Domestic Violence Bill. Most recent studies find that the situation remains little changed in the early 2000s, although much effort has been directed toward service improvement (see Taylor-Browne, 2001), so that a greater level of service user satisfaction could reasonably have been anticipated. In a very recent study for Women's Aid, named *Routes to Safety*, Cathy Humphreys and Ravi Thiara from the Centre for the Study of Safety and Well-being at the University of Warwick found, for example, that agency responses to women's help-seeking in response to domestic violence were very mixed (Humphreys and Thiara, 2002). While many of the 200 women and thirteen children who completed questionnaires or were interviewed had experienced positive responses overall, there was a large percentage who had been unhappy about the services they had received. Women in this recent study consistently recommended that what the users of services most need and value include the following: an immediate response; accurate information, advice and referral; a respectful and professional attitude; a proactive approach; and consistency across social divisions of ethnicity, class, sexuality and disability (ibid.: 119). While these recommendations related principally to the police, they were considered relevant across the board.

In the authors' study referred to throughout this book, the majority of the 112 women interviewed felt that their views were overlooked to a considerable extent by service providers and that their needs were not adequately met. They felt silenced, regarded as not important and unable to achieve the type of service and policy responses that they sought. Most felt they were powerless to influence the direction of policy or service development and they related accounts of inadequate or potentially dangerous responses by agencies, alongside some improved services. Forty-five per cent of the women we spoke with felt that they had not been believed by the agency approached. Gratifyingly, 58 per cent overall had nevertheless been assisted to feel and be safe. However, 42 per cent had continued to be unsafe and unprotected, sometimes over long periods of ineffective service intervention. Overall, only 19 per cent of interviewees had been asked what their own needs were by agencies approached for help and, in one of the study areas, this was as low as 3.7 per cent.

At the same time as frequently feeling silenced and excluded, many of the women interviewed thought that agency practice had indeed got better in various ways over recent years. Encouragingly, for 59 per cent of interviewees overall, there was a belief that services had substantially improved in the 1990s and 2000s, but, in one study area (not the same one referred to above), this figure was only 29 per cent. Improvements, where these had occurred, included increases in numbers of services and more understanding or sympathetic officers. The police were felt by the largest percentage of women to have improved the most, but the findings of the study in this respect were contradictory. Despite transformations in service in many areas, this research, like the earlier studies mentioned previously, found that police responses to domestic violence in the 2000s have continued to be uneven overall. A notable exception in our study was provided by domestic violence units and liaison officers. These were regarded very positively. In fact, almost all the improvements reported in the study were associated with these specialist units and officers, and relatively few with the uniformed general service, a vote of confidence in this type of dedicated provision. Importantly, however, specialist police domestic violence services are under threat of closure in some localities, or at least face reductions in staff or amalgamations into larger units, focusing on vulnerable persons, community safety or child protection/family violence, which can mean a dilution of expertise and of attention to violence against women.

Similarly, the *Routes to Safety* study, cited previously, found that many women victims had positive experiences of using the police, especially where specialist units had been involved (Humphreys and Thiara, 2002: 60). However, the study noted that positive responses from the police can depend on the woman being a 'good victim'. Once falling into the 'bad victim' category, perhaps by wanting to drop the case during prosecution or by remaining with their partners despite many incidents of violence, women interviewees in this study reported a variety of dismissive responses from the police. Overall, the positive responses reported were accompanied by an equal level of comments from women who had found that policing responses fell far short of their expectations (ibid.: 60).

While women respondents in our own study were most positive about the police changes, they also noted changes in other agencies. After the police viewed positively by 54 per cent, interviewees identified the most improvements within statutory agencies as being within housing at 41 per cent, while other statutory agencies scoring at markedly lower percentages. Social services came out at 29 per cent, for example, and the health service at 25 per cent. The courts and the Benefits Agency were the least impressive at 13 per cent and 12 per cent respectively, in terms of whether or not they had improved their responses to abused women. Given the importance of both financial support and legal remedies through either the criminal justice system or the civil law for women escaping domestic violence, these findings are particularly concerning.

Slightly different figures were found in relation to how much the agencies women had approached for help actually understood about the needs of abused women and children in relation to services. Again, these figures were extremely disappointing in relation to the courts and the Benefits Agency which scored positively for only 3.5 per cent and 4 per cent each all interviewees, although these figures were somewhat better for those who had actively used their services in the recent past, at 10 and 8 per cent respectively. The police overall scored only 28 per cent overall, but this figure rose to 40 per cent for those who had recently used the service directly. These findings indicate that women may find that these agencies sometimes give a better service in practice now than they might expect them to do based on previous experience. A stunning result was achieved, once again, by the specialist police domestic violence liaison officers at 96 per cent, and refuge organisations came in at 98 per cent for those who had directly used the service recently.

Thus, in this research, refuge and outreach organisations scored by far the best in terms of satisfaction with services received, with positive comments from women service users across the board. Recent work in the 2000s has confirmed this situation, not only as regards refuge provision but also in relation to women's outreach and support services (see, e.g. Kelly and Humpheys, 2000). For example, the *Routes to Safety* study analysed the effectiveness of two types of outreach services. One type provides support for women who have lived in refuges, while the other is for women who have never used such a service (Humphreys and Thiara, 2002). Within a very wide range of outreach services and considerable variations in the effectiveness and extent of provision, women service users generally found the service helpful and appreciated meeting with other women. Children's views were also sought during this study. The children interviewed had positive feelings about the outreach service they had attended, rated it highly and, in some cases, felt that their relationships with their mothers had improved as a result of attending (ibid.: 36).

However, this encouraging response to specialist service provision by women's refuge, advocacy and support projects needs to be viewed against the background of chronic underfunding of these voluntary sector organisations. It is doubtful that this will be adequately addressed by the Supporting People initiative which is funding refuges from 2003 (DETR *et al.*, 1998), since this will provide resources primarily for housing provision rather than for support needs, despite the stated commitment of some of the new officers within this initiative to both refuge and outreach provision.

Thus, in summary, improvements are ongoing across the board, but refuge services are still underfunded, and survivors in the authors' study who had used other agencies identified continuing gaps in provision that had left them vulnerable and unsafe. We turn now to further findings from the study to discuss why the involvement of service users and other domestic violence survivors needs to be an integral part of all policy development, not something suddenly thought of and 'added on' at the last minute, as appears often to be the case. We will then move on to debate what actually happens as regards such involvement in reality.

Chapter 5

How much do agencies listen to domestic violence survivors?

This chapter discusses the extent of agency commitment to domestic violence survivor consultation and participation, and considers how much the views of women experiencing violence are heard – and, more importantly, listened to – by professionals. We begin by discussing why user involvement needs to be integral to policy-making and service provision, and then look at how much agencies, including statutory services and inter-agency forums, involve domestic violence survivors at the moment, leading on to a consideration of women's movement projects and survivor participation. We conclude by looking at the way that workers in all sectors often view abused women as unworthy participants while they are still 'in the experience'.

In investigating these issues and in looking at empowerment and the raising of the voices of abused women, we can learn, as discussed briefly in Chapters 2 and 3, from the sometimes inspiring contributions of other service user movements which have self-organised over recent years to challenge poor or discriminatory services. Thus, a key tool – both in effectively listening to, and in theorising from the views of service users – is the body of literature on service user involvement more generally. As we have discussed, the movements concerned have campaigned for better services and have also produced guidance on how to conduct consultation effectively (see, for example, Lindow, 1994; Department of Health, 1996a). The disability movement and the movement of psychiatric service survivors have been particularly active in this regard, and have also theorised responses to social issues from the perspectives of those involved (for disabled people, see Swain *et al.*, 1993; Campbell and Oliver, 1996; Priestley, 1999; for psychiatric service survivors, see Barker and Peck, 1987; Chamberlin, 1988; Brandon, 1991; Sayce, 1999).

Why should user involvement be integrated into service development?

As we argued in theoretical terms in Part 1, the contributions of these user movements and the increased recent attention to the views and needs of people using services have led to broad conceptualisations of the empowerment of users in relation to a wide range of public services, including child protection, community care, housing and health (Hastings *et al.*, 1996; Means and Smith, 1996; Barnes and Warren, 1999; Barnes *et al.*, 1999). Using these ideas, cogent arguments as to the importance of involving service users in service provision and delivery can be elaborated in relation both to the importance (and frequent ignoring) of social movements, and to the empowerment of those who have suffered disadvantage and exclusion in relation to general notions of citizenship and community (see Barnes and Oliver, 1995; Barnes, *et al.*, 1996). In theory, greater accountability of services can be achieved through participatory democracy, although this often does not happen in reality (Braye, 2000; Cull and Roche, 2001). Community development, for example, has a long history but has often failed to promote dialogue and meaningful involvement (Barnes, 1997). The development of service user movements and the empowerment of users themselves can be an antidote to these failures.

There are further convincing reasons for listening to service users. Broadly speaking, the positive practical outcomes of user involvement can be argued to outweigh by far the attendant difficulties in terms of achieving more focused and responsive services and more democratic policy-making. Many service user movements have suggested that, in general, user participation is an essential and basic component of good policy-making, in order to regulate and to 'keep an eye on' service provision (Barnes *et al.*, 1999). In this argument, it is not an option that policy-makers may or may not engage in, depending on their level of personal or professional commitment but, rather, a fundamental matter. Along these lines, within the domestic violence field specifically, we would assert from our study that the involvement of women who have experienced abuse in policy and service development needs to be an integral element, built into the process and properly funded so that it becomes possible and practical to achieve it.

There are many justifications to support this assertion. An important one is that user involvement and consultation is now officially and legally required, as we noted in Chapter 3. It is beginning to be common practice in many types of service provision to engage in the routine seeking of the views of service users in relation to customer satisfaction and service evaluation. On both an operational and a strategic level for policy-makers, user consultation is now necessary as part of the legislative and policy dictates that agencies need to meet in terms of targets and performance indicators (Hague *et al.*, 2002). It has become a mainstream issue in this sense, placing a legal duty of consultation on all designated authorities. In relation to domestic violence specifically – a hidden crime and one that has been traditionally under-documented – it can be very helpful that there is so much official and government emphasis currently on seeking user views, although it is important to make use of this new situation in a creative and effective way. Disturbingly though, while rhetoric about the issue has become widespread, most service user movements in a variety of fields report that concrete strategies have been lacking, often leading, as we saw in Chapter 3, to ineffective or cosmetic outcomes, or to a bureaucratic type of consultation with no subsequent effect on policy or change (Barnes and Oliver, 1995; Cooper et al., 1995). As part of this process, tactics used by project managements to accept what service users say when it suits them, but to use various strategies to de-legitimise them when it does not, have also been widely reported, as noted above (Barnes et al., 1999).

Being forced to engage in consultation by government, while very useful if carried out effectively, results of course in a 'top-down' type of process, as we discussed in Part 1. From a more 'bottom-up' position, getting managers and policy-makers to listen to people's voices 'on the ground' is likely to spread involvement locally through community participation (Beresford and Croft, 2001). At best, this can lead to self-advocacy and to real accountability of policy and services to those being consulted. Thus, the involvement of users of services can be seen to be important in terms of improving local processes of participation and accountability. Such mechanisms are also essential so that better, more efficient, outcomes can be achieved. User participation for abused women can result in the provision of services which are safe, proactive, sensitive and respectful, leading to increased customer satisfaction all round. Services and policy become more effectively focused on expressed needs, and these needs can inform and be built into both present provision and future planning. Thus, user involvement enables services and policy development in both the statutory and voluntary sectors to be kept on track, and to be subjected to – and able to withstand – user scrutiny. Without abused women's voices to provide a 'reality check', official responses can result in professional interventions that are cut off from what is really needed. Sometimes, for example, lengthy policy documentation and implementation on domestic violence can take place, taking much time but resulting in little change (Home Office, 2000; Hague et al., 2001a).

Overall, the single most important performance measure for any agency or practitioner to apply in working with domestic violence is: 'Will my intervention leave this woman and her children in greater safety or in greater danger?' The issue of giving survivors a voice, both individually and collectively, revolves around the fact that they almost always apply safety as their overarching criterion and that they are likely to be able to make judgements about it more knowledgeably and skilfully than professionals alone. They also ask the searching questions about system failures – why the victim was not adequately protected, why the perpetrator was not held accountable, why effective services were not provided. It is these questions which help multi-agency domestic violence forums to become more than talking shops and individual agencies to make radical improvements in their services.

Thus, user participation results in better value for money and more effective use of resources as services can be tailored more efficiently to need. It contributes to improved liaison with survivors and with the women's advocacy agencies that represent them, and guards against the possibility of cosmetic or inappropriate responses and of policies and practice going wrong. It can also demonstrate where implementation of services can be best focused by exposing any gaps between what is meant to happen and what actually does. Vitally, it also contributes on a personal level to individual and collective empowerment for abuse survivors.

During our study, these positive outcomes were identified many times as anticipated possibilities by both professionals and women who had used services. The positives were suggested so far to outnumber the negatives that it can be hard to understand why consultation (at the least) with domestic violence survivors is not standard practice. In summary, the anticipated benefits included improved and more effective services and policies that would be responsive to abused women's stated needs; the avoidance of 'talking' or 'smokescreen' responses from professionals; increased accountability and democracy in terms of service provision; and the empowerment of abuse survivors. A further bonus is seen as increased liaison between, on the one hand, service providers, local and central government agencies and the statutory and voluntary sectors, and, on the other, abused women and the agencies (women's support and refuge services) that represent them.

Mainstreaming: survivor participation in multi-agency forums and statutory agencies

So, we might well ask whether the positive outcomes associated with service user participation, and the compelling reasons for engaging in it, have been taken on board in the domestic violence field. Is it possible to locate some practical examples of abused women service users being viewed as a powerful user group in their own right, as we theorised in Chapter 2? Now that provision for abused women is more widely available, it is important to know whether service delivery has been directly and deliberately informed by women's voices and the extent to which domestic violence agencies and policy-makers have accepted the importance of listening actively to what survivors of violence have to say. The answers to these questions are understandably complex, and vary to some extent from agency to agency and from locality to locality, across all the different types of agencies involved. Some overall observations can, however, be made to inform more detailed analysis.

In terms of overarching understandings, then, it can be seen from the discussion up to this point that there are two, contrasting, situations at play in regard to consultation with women who have been abused. The first of these is that, until now, women survivors of domestic violence have typically reported unhelpful responses, poor services and the experience of being silenced or stigmatised by statutory agencies which may also engage in cosmetic or ineffective consultation, if they engage in any at all (Hague *et al.*, 2001). The second is that, in this field of work, unlike some others, there is a wider activist movement championing survivors in general and trying to raise the voices of abused women and their children, which has pioneered the way (Schechter, 1982; Hanmer and Itzen, 2000).

In the improving situation currently, it is of some use to ask how much agencies in the former category are being influenced by the latter. In the rest of this chapter, we will discuss the extent to which agencies and forums have taken on the issue of participation by survivors. We will couch this discussion within a consideration of whether inter-agency forums and the new services and statutory responses of the 2000s have taken a cue from women's refuge and advocacy services in terms of an empowering engagement with those using the services, or whether the influence has been more the other way round. Dealing first with the mainstream response, then, our study was able to analyse how much domestic violence survivors are consulted by statutory and voluntary sector agencies and how much these services, projects and policies are accountable (in any way at all) to women service users themselves. It will come as little surprise that the short answer to both these questions is 'not much'.

From both the literature to date and from the study reported here, it appears that much of the recent mainstream response to domestic violence has focused on policy development which, though often creative and dedicated, has not necessarily been marked by involving or consulting women who have experienced abuse directly. In the last couple of years, there has been a belated, and far from universal, recognition that abused women's views constitute the single most important element in the evaluation of perpetrators' programmes (Mullender and Burton, 2001) as we noted in Chapter 2. However, apart from some of this provision, and with the notable exception of women's refuge and support services, it seems that most domestic violence projects and inter-agency forums do not involve abused women directly (see Mullender and Hague, 2001).

A tendency for statutory agencies to 'take over' multi-agency domestic violence forums has been identified in research studies, and women's advocacy and outreach projects themselves have sometimes been marginalised within top-down policy development (Hague *et al.*, 1996; Home Office, 2000; Kelly and Humphreys, 2001). Encouragingly, our own study found that almost all domestic violence forums and other services do believe, in theory, that the involvement of women's refuge and advocacy groups is an important priority, although the practice could be rather different. In focus group-type workshops run by our study, the point was often made that, in reality, both domestic violence forums and higher level partnership group-ings sometimes overlooked and excluded Women's Aid and other women's advocacy organisations – let alone groups of survivors. Just keeping Women's Aid on board was hard enough. These findings confirmed those of the previous national study of multi-agency initiatives mentioned earlier (Hague *et al.*, 1996). Workshop members who were workers in refuges spoke of not being invited to meetings and so not knowing when user involvement or consultation exercises were about to take place, and then finding their views sidelined in resulting policy reviews or recommenda-tions. Sometimes, organisations like Women's Aid were viewed as just one organisation among many of equal weight (including some which worked only very occasionally with domestic violence). In fact, however, women's organisations are frontline providers of key importance. Domestic violence forums and agencies need to be cognisant of this central role and of the importance of women's refuge and advocacy services in developing policy and practice. Where Women's Aid and other women's organisations are struggling to stay involved, it can be even harder for the voices of domestic violence survivors and service users to be heard.

In the study, it was clear that some multi-agency forums do seriously attempt to engage in good practice as regards both the involvement of women's services and consultation with survivors. These forums may contain dedicated officers from a variety of agencies who are strongly committed to improving responses to domestic violence. Some are willing to experiment with new ideas and to try sensitively to reach women service users and seek out their views in a careful and systematic way. On the other hand, as far as wholeheartedly engaging with service users in order to shift power – actual, real power – and decision-making in their direction is concerned, the number of inter-agency forums and other domestic violence projects trying to open themselves and their procedures in order to do this was minimal. Thus, we were able to discern a difference between workers in forums and agencies who were willing just to consult and those who were keen to take the involvement of abused women further.

As discussed in Part 1, progress within service user movements in general began to be made in the 1990s in the form of an important, user-driven transition from notions of 'having a say' to having 'greater control' (User-Centred Services Group, 1993) and making services 'user-led' (Morris, 1994), but was then somewhat overtaken theoretically by postmodern ques-tionings of both the possibility and legitimacy of collective action for change (Servian, 1996). It is only recently that ideas of celebrating diver-sity and difference within a collectivity have once more made user-led change appear feasible (Leonard, 1997; Batsleer and Humphries, 2000). It is clearly important to harness these more sophisticated notions of power as a counter to sometimes naive good intentions in policy and professional quarters (or equally naive rejections of the belief that any form of representation is possible). However, our study was able to identify only one or two practical examples where domestic violence agencies or multi-agency forums attempted to share real decision-making power or tried to be directly accountable to abuse survivors. More often, they engaged in consultation exercises (useful though these could be), if they took on the issue at all. There are currently a very few examples of sensitive methods being developed to involve, or at best to devolve power to, women service users, but many agencies in the domestic violence field continue to admit to a major shortfall between their rhetorical statements or wish-list and their actual achievements in giving women survivors of violence real influence (Hague *et al.*, 2001, 2002).

Domestic violence, however, is a complex, human issue. Its complexity means that answers to questions are rarely straightforward. In reflecting on the extent of the impact of survivor voices on service and policy development, it is important to remember and constantly to reaffirm that these voices are not solely those of women who are using, or have previously used, services. Rather, women who have experienced domestic violence are also present within almost all professional responses. Women who are themselves abuse survivors are represented among policy-makers and other professionals throughout the field, and have often taken a leading role in developing services. Thus, even if there is no machinery in place to consult service users or ex-users, the voices of abused women are in fact present. It is important to be clear about this significant issue, as discussed in Part 1, and about the fact that domestic violence survivors are represented throughout every level of society and are not limited to those who have used services. For example, multi-agency forums to address domestic violence continue to be much encouraged by government, as we have discussed (Home Office, 1999, 2000), and it is certain that survivors of abuse are represented on almost all of them. Many women professionals who have personal experiences of abuse take an active part, driving the work of the forums forward. Some may choose not to reveal their own past abuse while others refer actively to it, not as something belittling but as a way of pushing others to be proactive on the issue. One professional whom we interviewed in our study strongly stated her position as follows (although she also believed that further consultation would be beneficial):

> Well I object to being asked 'does the [forum] have ways of consulting survivors'. I'm a survivor and I don't mind who knows it and I'm the chair so they have to listen, don't they.
>
> (Chair of domestic violence forum)

It is service users, though, who are in the best position to comment on services received. Overall in our study, only 12 per cent of survivor interviewees had experience of domestic violence forums taking notice of service user views. However, almost all interviewees, both women who had experienced violence and agency representatives, felt that it was very important that they should do so, indicating a general willingness to address this issue in the future. From 258 responses from organisations across the country, it could be seen that the majority of forums wanted to involve survivors, even if few are currently doing so. It was also evident in our study that, while many particularly wanted to consult service users, they were often less clear about engaging in the next part of the process in terms of moving on from doing the consultation itself to making it a real part of the policy-making process. In the words of one forum member, delivered with a sardonic smile and a shrug, multi-agency forums were often 'keen on making policies but less keen on bringing agency policies down to the "real, the *raw*"'. Some interviewees, both service users and agency workers, felt that inter-agency forums and individual agencies made consultation difficult almost deliberately and hung on to their own powerful positions:

> Agencies and forums erect barriers (physical, procedural, emotional, practical, deliberate, unconscious etc.) to survivors being part of meetings and decision-making processes.
> (Officer from a multi-agency forum)

In total, 80 per cent of the women survivors themselves whom we interviewed believed that domestic violence survivors should be able to participate in, or contribute to, multi-agency forums and domestic violence services as automatic practice and right. The evidence of the study in general was that women who have experienced domestic abuse believe that, if practice were informed by their feedback and views, more efficient and cost-effective provision would result. In all the data collected, service user consultation and the development of policies that devolve some power and influence to domestic violence survivors were believed to offer a constructive way forward in the development of domestic violence forums, policies and services.

Specifically as regards consultation, the initial stage of any user participation programme, some multi-agency forums had developed innovative ways of carrying it out (which are further discussed in Chapters 8, 9 and 10), including domestic violence survivors' forums, focus groups and structured representation through Women's Aid. Some of these have the potential to move on from solely consultation to more comprehensive user involvement. These committed attempts need to be acknowledged and publicised in order to provide guidance and ideas for others (even while recognising that many forums have not taken on the issue at all as yet). A number of multi-agency forums approached in our study systematically consulted existing women's groups (for example, one London Borough worked directly and consistently over time with separate groups for Arabic-speaking women, refugee women, refuge users and African Caribbean and Asian women). In other cases, women who were, or who represented, survivors joined the organisation to assist with specific projects, or were consulted about a one-off piece of policy development (for example, planning services on a particular council estate).

Overall, though, under half of inter-agency forums consulted survivors in our study. Further, in some cases the consultation was extremely sketchy or was something that forums said they were in the process of doing but hadn't fully done yet. In others, the consultation consisted merely of needs-led surveys, rather than direct involvement, although still others had taken it forward in committed, careful and effective ways. In interpreting these findings overall, however, it should also be noted that a possible element of 'over-claiming' was observed, in that domestic violence inter-agency forums generally claimed that they had a better record in consulting women service users than women's refuge and outreach projects in their localities suggested they did.

As regards actual participation in the forum's structure, rather than consultation, the figures were somewhat different. Seventeen per cent of the forums nationwide whom we approached during our study involved survivors as members, and 15 per cent did so within their management structure, although it was not always clear whether these figures referred to service users and ex-users (in which case they seem quite high) or to survivors more generally (in which case, conversely, they seem rather low). Overall, the picture was constantly changing. This situation of change is partly because domestic violence forums themselves alter all the time and may not have a recognisable structure in any case, and partly because they lack statutory weight, unlike, for example, Area Child Protection Committees (ACPCs). As a result, they have no established resource base that could be drawn on to finance user consultation exercises. They may also be dominated by agencies that are unused to working collaboratively with service users.

Turning now to direct statutory and other services, our study found that, where they involved users at all, they did so less systematically than either refuge and outreach projects or domestic violence forums. None of the statutory or voluntary sector projects interviewed in the study, outside women's refuge, advocacy and support organisations, had any policies at all in place as regards direct access for users and ex-users to management and policy-making. Although there were examples of good practice and of attempts to involve service users and ex-users here and there, the over-riding view in the statutory sector (with some exceptions who were often local authority equality and other specialist officers and police domestic violence liaison officers) seemed to be that women who have experienced domestic violence deserve pity and protection.

It must be said that, in general, individual agencies did quite often make a stab at consultation, but frequently of the most rudimentary kind. They might, for example, consult their service users through exit questionnaires evaluating services received and through user surveys. At best, such evaluations and user feedback can then be helpfully fed into planning and development decisions about improving the service in the future. They can be most useful if operated systematically and if the agency concerned takes notice of, and acts upon, the results. Using the police as an example, it was clear from our study that police services use well-established mechanisms for gauging victim satisfaction with services received, but these do not appear to be well embedded in relation to domestic violence or necessarily to feed into wider consultative strategies (Mullender and Hague, 2001). None of the police domestic violence units in our study consulted their users in a wider way, except very informally (although some police services have advisory groups, including abuse survivors). We found few examples of statutory agencies involving service users in a more systematic or influential way to assist with policy development, apart from policy reviews or partnership plans and audits which generally require user input and had, in some cases, engaged in substantial consultation.

Between 29 and 32 per cent of our women interviewees believed that the views of abused women were taken more seriously by some of the new specialist domestic violence services in the statutory and voluntary sectors than by traditional services like housing departments. In general, these types of specialist provision were regarded very favourably in terms of consultation and involvement of service users. Current examples include the 'One stop shops' that have been established in various local authorities. The work of one of the pioneers of this approach, Ambassador One Stop Project in Croydon, in which women who have experienced violence take an active part in providing services, is discussed in Chapter 10. (The project is now named the One Stop Partnership.) There are so few specialist women's projects of this type, however, that we were unable to collect meaningful statistics from them, but it appears that they all consult women survivors whenever they can. This includes many of the projects currently being funded by the Home Office Crime Reduction Programme on Violence against Women.

Some of the abuse survivors and domestic violence workers with whom we talked in our study, in a variety of agencies and forums, had been developing survivor consultation and involvement strategies for some years and had much rich experience of what happens on the ground. The majority of these inter-agency respondents who had substantial amounts of expertise in developing effective consultation confirmed that domestic violence service users and their representatives (for example, women's refuge and support or advocacy organisations) were frequently marginalised and silenced in multi-agency work more generally. These experienced respondents made a case that satisfactory service and policy development can only occur when representation and some form of informal accountability have become:

> an integral and accepted part of the work, but few forums currently understand this on a real, 'felt and lived' level. It is crucial that user involvement and consultation is not just a trendy idea but is translated into policy, so that its raison d'être is to lead to action and change, not just to look good.
>
> (Multi-agency forum co-ordinator)

From their direct experience, they had learned the importance of concrete change and action, rather than fashionable consultation on its own.

Survivor participation in women's refuge, support and outreach services

Within the wide range of agencies now involved in domestic violence work, women's organisations are the most likely to view user participation as integral to what they do. Confirming the findings of many previous studies (for an overview, see Mullender and Hague, 2000, 2001), women's refuge and outreach projects in our own study had the best record, not only of providing sympathetic specialist services as discussed in the last chapter, but also of consulting and involving women and children using these services (although they often did so in a less systematic way than in the earlier days of the women's refuge movement). Service users and service providers within Women's Aid have always interacted together in a non-traditional way, attempting to be realistic about the power differentials between them, but also breaking down those differentials wherever possible.

Women residents and ex-residents attend regional and national meetings and conferences of the Women's Aid federations, for example, and frequently speak out about their experiences at events and feed their views into the organisation in various ways. Refuges and women's support organisations conduct many surveys and pieces of research to ascertain the views and needs of women experiencing domestic violence in general or using refuge services. The federations also contribute to, and have taken a pioneering role in, electronic consultation through the Internet (as further discussed later and in the Epilogue). Overall, survivors of violence and women using services have a high profile in Women's Aid, as compared with people using the services provided by most other voluntary sector agencies.

Table 5.1 Percentage of inter-agency forums and refuge services saying they
           involved service users (N = 258)

	Refuge services (%)	Inter-agency forums (%)
Women consulted	90	40
Women having influence over policy	77	36
Women having real power to contribute to decisions and policy	30	26

Table 5.1 compares the extent to which inter-agency forums and refuge organisations in our study consulted with service users and ex-users and compares this figure both with the percentage where women in these situations had some influence over policy-making, and with the figure where they had real power to participate in decision-making, according to agency representatives. Overall, 90 per cent of refuges reported consulting with their women residents and other survivors, an encouraging figure. By contrast, only 40 per cent of inter-agency forums across the country consulted with women service users. For all of these agencies and forums, even though it was a self-report survey, there was a precipitous decrease in percentages between those who solely consulted and those in which abused women were reported to exert a measure of real decision-making power, with those where service users had some influence over policy being in the middle.

These figures confirm what perhaps could have been predicted. Whereas a very high percentage of refuges and almost half of forums directly consulted domestic violence survivors in some way, a smaller percentage would be expected to involve survivors in a way that enables them to have some actual influence over policy and service direction. This was the case both for refuges, at 77 per cent of women having influence, and for inter-agency forums at only 36 per cent. Importantly though, while women users were far more often consulted and given influence in refuge groups than in domestic violence forums, there was little difference between them in terms of service users having any real power to participate actively in decision-making about the project. Refuge organisations scored 30 per cent here, and forums 26 per cent. This is a telling finding for refuge services, which often take pride in their principles of democratic sharing and of listening and empowerment as regards their service users. Admittedly, though, power is a difficult matter to categorise, and our informants may have been interpreting it in different ways in different agencies. Also, it may be a near impossible task to involve users and ex-users in actual decision-making more substantially within a moderately conventional service organisation (as opposed to an advocacy project, for example). Nevertheless, refuge organisations might have been expected to score more highly here.

Activist women's projects have always had general policies to empower abused women and their children which have often been carried out in practical, down-to-earth ways, and this continues. But, in the study reported here, the qualitative evidence was that Women's Aid and other refuge and support organisations were perhaps less able to involve their residents and ex-residents than they had been in the past, when it was very common for ex-users of the service to apply for jobs or to join the support group (the previous, more informal, name for what is now more often known as the management committee). This kind of involvement continues to a considerable extent, but somewhat less frequently than previously. Thus, rather than women's services influencing statutory bodies and new domestic violence projects to involve users and ex-users more, the influence has perhaps operated the other way round to some extent. Rather than statutory services becoming more participative, women's refuge organisations and support projects appear to have become somewhat less so (although they have influenced statutory services positively in abused women's favour in many other ways). Many refuge services now involve service users less in their management and operation than they did formerly, at least in terms of women residents being able to participate in policy-making within the agency.

This development is partly an inevitable result of the enormously increased amount of monitoring, target-setting and paperwork that now afflicts Women's Aid as much as it does all other agencies. Participating in multi-agency and partnership initiatives has also added greatly to workloads (Harwin, 1999). These factors mean that time is limited and there can be a demand for specific skills and qualifications which ex-residents may not have. In general, the work done may be divided up between staff members along more hierarchical lines than in the past, and the overall employment structures currently in use in refuge organisations are often now less collective than they used to be (Hague et al., 2001). One woman who had both lived and worked in a refuge had this to say:

> It has changed so much. Before, you could get a job in the refuge as a survivor or go to the support group. It upsets me to think about how much it has changed.

> (Woman interviewee)

The trend towards 'professionalisation' and the demands of funders for a more managerial approach frequently cut across commitments to collaborative or participative structures within women's organisations. On a general level, it has been observed that projects tend to become less radical, and that innovatory dynamism is sometimes lost, as a response to main-streaming and professionalisation, although Women's Aid retains its critical edge. Over the years, there have been many debates about such issues in terms of the relationship between the women's movement and the state, and the possible co-optation of the former when the latter gets involved (see, e.g., Lovenduski, 1993; Hague and Malos, 1998). Our study adds some fuel to these debates in terms of the price of mainstreaming on activism in many (but by no means all) women's projects.

During our study, 40 per cent of refuge groups had residents' rights poli-cies in operation, although more of these are being developed all the time. In just 24 per cent, current residents could attend management meetings, despite a previous commitment throughout the refuge movement (particu-larly evident in the 1970s and 1980s) to collectivity in this respect. This was perhaps always a rather cosmetic commitment in that current residents could rarely participate in real decision-making, so often had no role at the meetings they attended. Their presence, though, meant that they were informed about, and involved in, what was going on within the organisa-tion. They often felt more important and respected, simply by being invited.

Of course, in the early stages of trying to escape their abusers, the last thing many survivors need is to be asked to attend meetings and groups, as 71 per cent of the women we interviewed pointed out. It can also be argued that it is good practice to maintain management functions separately from forums for service users in order to avoid a loss of clarity and the emergence of potentially messy or unprofessional situations. An alterna-tive might be to engage in formal representation processes, as is common practice elsewhere, with a quota of service users attending to represent the views of everyone else. However, overall, it appears that there has been a loss in many refuge groups in terms of the lessening of the ability both to challenge traditional ways of running the organisation and to do things in different, and exciting, new ways.

The situation as regards ex-service users in Women's Aid is different again. In 52 per cent of the refuges in our study, ex-residents (unlike resi-dents) not only attended but sat formally on management committees and, in many cases, took official positions in the project (for example, as chair). Most refuges have policies that this is only possible after a certain time period has elapsed to allow the ex-resident concerned to move on from her own personal crisis so that she can take a more general view of the overall issues, as befits a manager. This strategy has been developed over many years of practice. For example, some refuge groups have a policy that ex-users can only join the management committee after all the women who were their friends when they were in the refuge have left, which would appear to be sensible practice in terms of confidentiality and avoiding inevitably vested interests. Others have a time period of typically six months which must elapse. However, if women experiencing abuse are willing to participate earlier, our study found that there may be room for a more flexible approach, cognisant of the complex emotional difficulties involved. Rigid policies are likely to have a negative effect on those women who are ready to participate earlier, whereas their participation in refuge operation and management can be a very positive personal experience, as many survivors have testified over the years within Women's Aid. Furthermore, a blanket policy will never be right for everyone, particularly in respect of an issue that can have a long-term impact. It may be how a woman is supported in surviving her experiences that counts, rather than a simple lapse of time. Women's refuges are currently in the process of revisiting some of these difficult but challenging issues.

On an operational level, rather than a managerial one, on the other hand, more than half the refuge projects which we consulted during our study involved residents in the actual running of the project. Women took responsibility within the project itself, even if not in the management structure, and participated in day-to-day decisions in a variety of ways, including handling admissions, deciding on internal policies, and making decisions and sharing ideas through house meetings. Refuge services also often involve women residents and other survivors in outward-looking work on awareness-raising, for example the design and production of leaflets and publicity materials (or in providing ideas for, and then choosing from, professionally produced designs). Women survivors from refuges are also involved in representing the organisation to external bodies and in training provision, both in contributing to the content of the training and also on occasion in participating in its delivery. Encouragingly, in our study, children could take a role in decision-making in 52 per cent of refuge groups and 69 per cent held children's meetings. These findings on children are supported by the independent findings of a recent mapping study of services for families where there is domestic violence, which found similar percentages (see Humphreys et al., 2000).

The Women's Aid federations have been working over the last ten years to improve the accountability and effectiveness of management and operational structures in refuge projects, and these developments have in some cases included mechanisms for consultation with service users. Consultation is included in Women's Aid Codes of Practice and in the performance indicators used. Overall, too, in almost all refuge groups consulted in our study, women who had experienced domestic violence were represented as professionals among volunteers, staff or management (whether or not they had revealed to colleagues what had happened to them in the past). Despite a diminishing of previous formal commitments to collectivity, refuge providers continue to offer an often creative engagement between women who have experienced domestic violence and those who have not.

Being 'in the experience'

A contentious issue was identified during our study about abused women who were still considered to be 'in the experience' of abuse and were therefore not taken seriously. All agencies appear to play into this. This includes statutory agencies who in the past have often displayed a patronising attitude to those who used their services but who may now be trying to leave that heritage behind, not always with great success (see, e.g. Humphreys and Thiara, 2002). It also includes, more surprisingly, some women's advocacy and support services. Being labelled as still being 'in the experience' relates to the way in which refuge groups may insist, as noted above, that ex-residents take a break from the organisation for a set time period after service use before being eligible to contribute to the management committee. In general, for all agencies, many workers appear to take the view, to varying degrees, that women service users are likely to be unreliable participants or informants, owing to emotional factors and unresolved trauma caused by the violence which they have experienced. Abused women are frequently, therefore, left out of consultation procedures, at least until their abuse is well in the past. Strategies of exclusion of this type can discriminate against some service users, and interviewees in one of the main study areas felt that the raw strength of survivor voices could be overlooked, while simultaneously recognising the complex emotional difficulties involved, which necessitate a particularly sensitive and flexible approach.

By labelling or 'constructing' survivors in this way, workers in all sectors in the domestic violence field sometimes unwittingly constrain and disempower those who are ostensibly being helped. When asked to talk in our study about why they thought this was, and how survivors could be involved more effectively in policy-making and the provision of domestic violence services, the same qualification (echoed by voluntary and statutory agency representatives alike) was often applied, although sometimes expressed slightly differently. Thus, women who had experienced violence were seen as rightfully involved, but not until they had 'moved on from the experience'. Ways of expressing this view included 'survivors have enough to deal with already' and 'they should not remind themselves' (quotes from agency representatives). Officers in both statutory and voluntary agencies were often similarly reticent, citing both lack of expertise among service users and ex-users, and lack of resources, as key factors in a regrettable situation.

Abused women often have much creativity to offer in terms of surviving abuse. Rather than recognising this, however, or seeing participation as a way in which domestic violence survivors might gain strength, confidence and control over their lives, workers in the field, ranging from statutory managers to some refuge workers, frequently took the opposite view. They appeared to feel that the experience of men's abuse rendered women so vulnerable and so much in need of protection (from a range of outside influences as well as from their abusers), that they were usually not able to engage in consultative and participative processes at all, at least in the short term. In the next section, this complex issue is discussed further, in terms of the empowerment of domestic violence survivors, on the one hand, versus, on the other, the silencing and stigma which they are frequently forced to endure.

Part 3

How to engage in survivor participation and consultation

Chapter 6

How to do it

Empowerment and stigma

> Something positive has come out of our sadness, out of our experiences, and others can learn from this.
>
> (Survivors from the Phoenix Group, City of Westminster)

Out of sadness, can come change. The women in the group quoted above are currently participating actively in the policy process, and their pain and experience are indeed leading to positive developments for other women in similar situations. They are clear that the best way to prevent domestic violence is to consult survivors of the violence. This statement was made to us several times in our research by a variety of different workers, agencies and abuse survivors. Who better to give meaningful information and to suggest possible solutions and effective responses to such violence than those who have had direct experience of it, working in tandem with policy-makers, practitioners and activists? However, this does not happen nearly as often as it should.

In Part 2, the frequent lack of consultation and participation strategies to involve survivors of abuse in the work of inter-agency forums and agencies was discussed. In order to correct this situation we need to ask what has to happen for abused women to be able to raise their own voices effectively and for these voices to be properly heard by policy-makers and service providers. In Part 3 then, we move on to discuss the 'how to' of user involvement in the domestic violence field. We address how, for example, to engage in survivor consultation and participation in a way that takes on the complexities involved, and which is meaningful, rather than merely cosmetic. We also discuss the practical methods that are currently being tried out, together with the positives and drawbacks of each. In doing this, we draw, as throughout this book, on the findings of our study and on the insights and lessons of the activist movement to empower women experiencing domestic violence. Thus, this is less an academic analysis than a practically oriented discussion to provide ideas, nuance and guidance for practitioners, activists and abused women themselves.

In the current chapter, we discuss ways of involving survivors in the policy process in general terms, and engage in a detailed consideration of stigma and the silencing effects of abuse, both of which need to be recognised and combatted in concrete ways as a basic foundation-stone of any practical survivor participation strategy. We then discuss the important issue of the collective and individual empowerment of abuse survivors that such strategies can facilitate, and end by considering the benefits of listening to abused women.

In terms of service user involvement in general in the domestic violence field, there are many different ways of seeking the views of survivors of violence and incorporating these into policy and practice. However, it is clear, as was discussed in the last section, that professionals in the field have only just begun to embark upon, and to explore, this challenging road. In various areas of the country, a few pioneers are currently experimenting with different approaches, and both workers and women using services are putting themselves on the line to try something new. In this endeavour, praise and recognition are due. One thing that is clear from the research we have undertaken is that the building of consultative methods and meaningful involvement for domestic violence service users is not an easy task. Achieving the accountability of services to users and shifting real power in their direction are massively harder. Even if consultation alone is considered, there are many thorny issues to be addressed and no one is yet sure of the best way to go about it.

It may be, in fact, that there is no 'best way'. We found in our research that methods and strategies vary, according to what is going on in the locality concerned. Thus, no single strategy for consultation or participation emerged as better than any other. Rather, approaches appear to depend on local circumstances and conditions, so that strategies which are effective in one area may not be so somewhere else, needing instead to be individually tailored. What will work where cannot necessarily be prescribed in advance.

Crucial factors which have an effect on whether accountability and user involvement ideas are likely to take hold in a locality include how widely services and domestic violence forums have been developed in the area concerned, together with the presence or absence of refuges and women's support services and also of key local personnel to take a pioneering role (see also Hague et al., 1996). The employment, within both refuges and the other service agencies dealing with domestic violence, of sometimes charismatic figures with a deep commitment to women survivors of abuse is often helpful, although willingness to give user involvement a try is perhaps more crucial. The issue needs champions to take it forward. Where service users, employees and managers are indeed willing to take the first steps, and where, in addition, activists are willing to support those who do so, real progress is possible.

Thus, active support for participation is required by organisations, both at a managerial strategic level and at an operational one, in order to make domestic violence user involvement work. Where such a commitment is made by managers as well as practitioners, it needs to operate on both a 'theoretical' and a practical level. In the study on which this book is based, though, it was clear that, while there was a wide commitment in principle among inter-agency domestic violence forums and agencies across the country to service user accountability and participation, few had much of an idea of how to do it in down-to-earth ways, nor, in almost all cases, were any available resources allocated.

One thing that has become clear to us as we have talked with those practically engaged in the enterprise around the UK is that approaches used may flower for a while and then may die away, to be replaced after a time, perhaps, by another method. Participants may be distressed when their efforts seem to have been of no avail, but such an outcome need not be regarded negatively. The fact that a strategy worked for a period of time is more important than its longevity. Peaks and troughs are experienced within attempts to engage in service user participation and community activism in all fields (see Lindow, 1995), as we noted in Chapter 3. But this tendency can be particularly important to acknowledge within domestic violence services due to the crisis nature of the work, the necessity for security and confidentiality, and the fact that abused women and children may need to be geographically mobile. Thus, things may change quite quickly. In one local area in which we worked in 1999–2000, for example, a particularly pioneering survivors' group had been a forerunner of its type but had not endured over time, as further discussed in Chapter 8. However, its legacy has enabled others to learn from the experience. The evidence from our research in relation to this experiment and to other ground-breaking attempts has led us to believe that the flowering should be celebrated, rather than leading to disillusion because of the possible subsequent dying away.

In general, then, involving domestic violence survivors can be a sensitive and difficult matter. If it is to be successful, overall strategic direction is needed within agencies, sensitively developed with the involvement of domestic violence survivors themselves wherever possible, accompanied by concrete procedures agreed by all concerned. Developing and operating such strategies and procedures can be a complex, and potentially painful, task. This is partly due to the distressing and often traumatic nature of the abuse that women are likely to have experienced and also to the need for safety issues to be paramount. We address these issues further in the next chapter but, first, we believe it is important to acknowledge that, when it works, survivor participation can be very moving and powerful for all involved and can be of great significance for policy development. If it is set up well, with attention to the sensitivities involved and with commitment and good planning and resources, the results can be extraordinary, according to the findings of our study. Women's lives and confidence can be transformed, and so can service provision and delivery:

> You can do something to give back some of the things you have learnt . . . and say, 'Look, it can be done' and make a contribution. People listen to me and I feel strong now and that I can help out other women. We all have to help each other, that's the only way to beat this thing. It's slow but we're getting there. . . . We're getting there. . . .
>
> (Interview with woman ex-service user)

Domestic violence survivors speaking out: stigma versus empowerment

Survivor participation can, then, be a powerful and passionate process and speaking out can have extraordinary results. Domestic violence, however, is not an easy issue to speak out about. Rather than the invigorating strengthening to which the woman quoted above alludes, the more common experience for abuse survivors is of being silenced, coupled with the possibility of being pathologised if you break the silence. In this section, we discuss these difficulties and ways of overcoming them through the empowerment, both of survivors individually, and of groups coming together collectively to challenge abuse. All attempts to develop survivor participation and accountability need to take on these issues as a fundamental and integral part of everything they do, and to do so consciously, sensitively and in practical 'real-life' ways, if they are to stand a chance of success. Stigma, silencing – and empowerment – are at the heart of the matter.

Stigma

Survivor involvement and empowerment cannot flourish if those involved, both professionals and service users, hold negative views about women who have experienced violence. However, this appears very often to be the case. In other arenas (see, for example, Aris *et al.*, 2003), we have argued that survivors of domestic violence may be stigmatised and deskilled by societal attitudes, and this may happen even within the very agencies that are most sympathetic to their situations, as discussed in the last chapter. Previous research has shown that, despite many recent improvements, there is widespread misunderstanding of the nature of domestic violence, not just among the general public, but also among workers in the statutory and other agencies to whom the majority of women experiencing abuse, and seeking help, turn for assistance and support (Smith, 1989; Hester and Pearson, 1998; Home Office, 2000). This lack of understanding has had serious consequences for survivors of such violence and their children in relation to access to services, and it has cost some women their lives. It has also silenced and stigmatised abused women within the commonly held view, to which we alluded at the end of the last section, that those who have experienced domestic violence somehow become less competent than those who have not. In our research, workers both in statutory agencies and in some refuge and advocacy organisations often seemed to impose stereotypes on survivors (either consciously or unconsciously) in such a way that they absorbed a sense of themselves 'as helpless paralysed victims who can't manage daily life' (quote from woman survivor). Such attitudes are clearly likely to militate against survivor participation strategies and will need to be carefully taken on as part of any implementation plan.

There are parallels to this situation in other fields, notably in the disability rights movement where the extent to which 'pity oppresses' has now been made clear and challenged. Activists in this movement reject ideas that present disabled people as being dependent and defined by their impairment (Wolf, 1993). Within the struggle to combat domestic violence, moves have also been made in this direction. However, many respondents in our study, both workers and service users themselves, saw survivors of violence as so adversely affected psychologically by their experience as to be both unreliable and incapable, at least temporarily, of participating in decision-making, as we have noted.

To some extent, the negative psychological effects are quite often real, at least for a time. But they are likely to be compounded by adverse messages, relayed often unconsciously by agencies and conveyed by those in a position to offer services and support. Interviewees talked of damaged job prospects, of low self-esteem, of avoiding reporting abuse and of editing their experiences to preserve themselves in a non-stigmatised situation because they knew how others regarded them.

A variety of women interviewees had these words to contribute: 'I didn't tell them it's domestic violence and they didn't ask'; 'I wanted to get a divorce by two years separation so as to gloss over the violence'; 'I wouldn't tell them the truth ... frightened of their reaction'; 'women don't want people to know; if they know they blame them'; 'I kept it quiet at the beginning'. Those who had experienced sexual abuse, in particular, found that the attitudes of others towards them often changed for the worse if they revealed it, so they usually edited it out. A few suspected some officials they had encountered of having a prurient interest, which had amplified the extreme personal embarrassment they already felt, and could even be compounded by sexual innuendo.

In these respects, it is plausible to argue that the identity of the survivors of domestic violence is not only reconstructed but, to use the term first pioneered by Erving Goffman in the 1960s, is 'spoiled' (Goffman, 1963). Stigma and the spoiling of identity in this way has the effect on an individual, in Goffman's words, of 'cutting him [sic] off from society and from himself so that he stands a discredited person facing an unaccepting world'

(ibid.: 19). Goffman's original and pioneering elaboration of this phenomenon (much developed by later writers) resonates with the reluctance of
many abuse survivors to participate in initiatives around domestic violence.
He asserts, for example, that someone with a stigma 'may perceive, usually
quite correctly, that whatever others profess, they do not really "accept"
him and are not ready to make contact with him on "equal grounds"' (ibid.:
7). Further, as Goffman notes:

> the standards he has incorporated from wider society equip him to be
> intimately alive to what others see as his failing, inevitably causing
> him, if only for moments, to agree that he does indeed fall short of
> what he really ought to be. Shame becomes a central possibility, arising
> from the individual's perception of one of his own attributes as being
> a defiling thing to possess.
>
> (ibid.: 7)

The gender-specific language, of course, belongs to the period in which it
was written, but, reframing it for the present day and in respect of abused
women, we can see how this process can damage how others see them and
how they may see themselves.

The belittling effect of viewing survivors of abuse in this way became
clear in the interviews and discussions with abused women which we
carried out. Some of those who were professionals themselves talked of
their input being diminished or marginalised if they disclosed their own
abuse, with the result that many of them had chosen not to do so, rather
than risk embarrassment and possible pity or voyeurism from colleagues.
If they were known to be domestic violence survivors, these workers
described how their objectivity and credibility were sometimes called into
question even in quite unrelated areas of their work.

A considerable percentage of the women we interviewed who were
service users were similarly reticent, and it is vital, if participation is to
work, for these views to be sensitively understood and addressed. Some
interviewees, for example, thought that survivors should actively participate in domestic violence forums – but not they, themselves. In Chapter 3,
the issue of not feeling qualified to participate in policy discussions was
discussed for service users more generally as a barrier to empowerment.
However, it was crucially compounded in this case by the impacts of the
violence. Those survivors we spoke to who were uneasy about participation were quick to talk of the disabling effects of experiencing abuse. While
some had become strong and vocal, many spoke of having been tainted by
the experience, and of the need to put it behind them and move on.

Thus, it can be particularly hard to identify yourself publicly in participation and consultation exercises as a survivor and to make yourself heard

(see Aris *et al.*, 2002). Some women in our study felt quite simply that they did not deserve to have a voice. These women, who had often suffered abuse over very many years, felt that their confidence and self-esteem were at too low an ebb and expressed anxieties about their own ability to contribute or to be seen as able to do so, as the following selection of quotes indicates: 'women need to get over the problems first'; 'survivors are seen as "silly women" '; and 'women are "not strong enough"'. Some interviewees were also doubtful in terms of their lack of information and skills. One suggested that: 'women would need a self-development course'; another that: 'there should be training and counselling for women who want to get involved'. Several were nervous of not being able to do what they were being asked:

> I don't know. I don't like the sound of it. Sounds frightening to me. Suppose you got it wrong, what would happen then? I think I'd rather leave it to them, they know what they're about.
>
> (Woman interviewee)

Empowerment

Yet, for women who have experienced abuse, the very process of survivor consultation and participation can be individually empowering, as we have noted, and can work against ideas and attitudes about stigma and spoiled identity. Where a group process is used, this empowering experience can also be a collective one. Such notions of empowerment very much resonate with the aims of Women's Aid and other women's organisations. The individual and collective empowerment of women has always been an important aim of the activist feminist movement since the early days (see, for example, Schechter, 1982; Dobash and Dobash, 1992; Davies, 1994; Hague and Malos, 1998) and, in the refuge movement, strong practical policies along these lines have been developed. These include a belief in the strength of women together and in the affirming nature of the notion that abuse is not the fault of the victim (Hague and Malos, 1998), as well as concrete policies to encourage group strengthening and career and life skills development.

Listening to abused women with dignity and respect and promoting their needs and views without judging them need to form the baseline of all strategies to develop survivor involvement, and are empowering in themselves. For example, current research in Women's Aid refuges (Abrahams, forthcoming) has demonstrated that active listening and respectful treatment by workers and the adoption of a non-judgemental attitude are crucially important if women are to rebuild confidence and self-esteem and to reconstruct their lives after abuse. Similarly, support groups, by their nature, if run supportively and sensitively, can enable abused women to build their strength and self-esteem. Members of a support group for women from minority ethnic communities whom we interviewed suggested that:

> Sharing experiences helps you – the group is very strengthening. It is hard emotionally to come to a group like this – to admit you've suffered violence and are going to a support group. But once you get over that and feel yourself here, it helps you, it makes you stronger and gives you friends and breaks your isolation. Women and children sticking together and helping each other – we love it!

Such experiences are supported by literature about resilience and coping strategies which emphasise the importance of both group support and personal involvement in planning processes and decision-making (Boushell, 1994). Grotberg (1997) and others have suggested, for example, that resilience and the ability of trauma victims to cope in the face of adverse circumstances can be encouraged by supportive interactions which foster autonomy, by the degree of development of individuals' own personal communication skills and by a sense that they are important and will be listened to and respected (see also Hester *et al.*, 2000; Mullender *et al.*, 2002). The particular work quoted here refers mainly to young people, but the same protective factors have been identified for adults. In terms of protection from debilitating and undermining aspects of intimate violence, the reality of being consulted about services and being regarded as important can have potentially transformative effects for abuse survivors.

Thus, for women who have experienced violence, the twin experiences of participating in support groups and of also being involved at the same time in decision-making about policy may reinforce each other, so that the empowering effect is likely to be magnified. It can be seen, then, that, at a personal level for women who have experienced abuse, survivor consultation and participation can contribute to individual empowerment. Women who are experiencing domestic violence are often excluded by their violent partners from decision-making and have been placed in a position of being unable to take meaningful control over their own lives. Taking part in consultation, or participating actively in a project, can counteract past abuse of this type. Women who may never have been listened to before, whose views may never have been regarded as important or worthy, are placed in a position where what they think is viewed as significant and helpful. The positive effects on self-esteem can scarcely be overemphasised.

Empowerment has been much debated (for a recent analysis, see, e.g. Barnes and Warren, 1999) and its positive features for communities, as well as for individuals, have been well elaborated (as opposed to its less grass-roots use in professional discourse to which we alluded in Chapter 3). In terms of groups rather than individuals, survivor groups that are engaged in consultation and accountability work with policy-makers and practitioners often experience collective empowerment, which can be a socially and politically significant outcome for previously excluded and disempowered women. Networks of support, friendships and the power of group support and cohesion are important factors here. Being part of decision-making in a group, being listened to collectively and having the power of the group behind you can build self-respect and confidence and enable those concerned to move forward in their lives in previously unimaginable ways.

However, overcoming stigmatisation and the resultant difficulties noted above may be hard to achieve in this way. Negative attitudes to domestic violence are difficult to shift, and pain and trauma may recur on an ongoing basis for survivors. This is a further reason for not excluding women who are 'in the experience'. In some ways, the experience never ends and arbitrary cut-off points are difficult to apply. Thus, in developing participation strategies, specific sensitivities and difficulties need to be recognised, named and negotiated, rather than being ignored, as so often happens if those involved are not familiar with the dynamics of domestic violence. Getting over the silencing effects of this type of violence and the possible impact on self-esteem are issues that need to be carefully taken on, if survivors are to be enabled to collaborate with agencies successfully. Similarly, there are many painful complexities and emotional issues involved in any disclosure of abuse. Such issues may be differently experienced as a result of cultural, ethnicity and class differences, and by the stressful effects of living as a migrant or as a member of a minority community in the UK (see Mama, 1996; Rai and Thiara, 1997). Any policy initiative on user participation must take on cultural matters and the reality of multiple discrimination and possible disadvantage.

In our study, the impacts of poverty and of living in socially excluded or marginalised conditions were also strong factors in impeding women's ability to participate in policy-making processes. Most of these personal and structural issues have implications in terms of identity and self-esteem. Additionally, because of the traumatic nature of domestic violence, there may be interpersonal conflict in ongoing consultative groups and problems with keeping such groups going over time. Further difficulties to be overcome that we identified in our study included the possible exploitation of unpaid members of the public by highly paid policy-makers and, vitally, issues of confidentiality and safety for women potentially at risk. These important matters are addressed throughout the remaining chapters.

In sum, then, our study found that there is a host of complexities to be addressed in order to enable women to raise their voices and to engage in individual and collective 'strengthening', which may include issues of identity, culture, discrimination, internal 'power' and self-image, and the shaming and debilitating effects of abuse. Where these can be dealt with sensitively and supportively, the experience can lead in powerful new ways both to individual empowerment for abused women and to collective empowerment through the strength of the group.

Listening to women who have experienced domestic violence

Survivors of domestic violence are currently making contributions to the policy process in a range of localities. The personal impact of survivor voices on policy-makers can be remarkable, and may add to the professional commitment of those policy-makers to instituting effective improvements in services, especially if they, themselves, are also survivors of abuse. The impact can also be remarkable for the survivors concerned, enabling them to contribute directly and in a constructive way to service and policy development, building on their own experiences. In our study, many women who had previously used services told us that they felt proud to give something back, to show their gratitude for the help they had received and to do what they personally could to assist other women. Two women had this to say:

> By working on domestic violence later, as a volunteer or worker, you can give back a bit of power and help to other women. Don't do it too soon – it would be too upsetting. Go away and come back to it. You need to heal first before you can help others.

> It helps to give a role model – I've survived, so can you.

Thus, when abused women join together to speak out, the emotional power of what they may say can be salutary for professionals. Many to whom we spoke expressed how moving they found such experiences, as the following member of an inter-agency forum described:

> The women provide real experience; their testimonies to the forum are very powerful and prevent our meetings becoming professional talking shops or purely academic. We couldn't stay on course without them.

However, as women ex-service users move away from service use and become accustomed to participating in service and policy development, some policy-makers and practitioners we interviewed felt that this emotive power had become muted by what they saw as professionalisation. In other words, as domestic violence survivors become accustomed to policy work, they begin to behave and think like the professionals they may previously have criticised. This issue was discussed in Chapter 3 as a general problem which has to be confronted and overcome by service user movements in terms of the possibility of losing impetus and integrity. However, while in our study we found a couple of examples of abuse survivors becoming demanding to work with as professionals, as one might expect in any situation, we uncovered few cases of professionalisation damaging women's commitment to the cause. Rather, the reverse was true in that ex-service users who had become workers in the system often brought renewed energy and understanding to the project in question. On occasion, of course, there may be some truth in the observation that ex-service users can begin to think like policy-makers and to curtail their demands accordingly. However, those survivors we interviewed who had considerable amounts of later professional experience in participation work told us that they felt this experience had facilitated their contributions, rather than detracting from them. They had been able to use their abilities in a more effective way through learning about the policy process.

Many women use survivor participation and consultation as a stepping stone to developing their own careers as volunteers or trained workers. The Women's Aid Federation of England has developed training courses for women service users, for example. NVQ courses in domestic violence now exist, some run in conjunction with refuge organisations, through which women service users or ex-users can gain qualifications which may then provide access to further training opportunities. Other courses (for example social work qualifying courses) may also offer possible avenues for career development, with eligibility to apply assisted by participation in consultation exercises and volunteer work by users or ex-users in the management or operation of projects.

It remains true that, whether or not professional changes of this type are facilitated for the women involved, many domestic violence survivors who have experience of working with agencies have given breadth and depth to policy responses by speaking out, and some have done so in powerful ways that have had strong effects, both for themselves and for the service in question. One woman said to us:

> I do what I can. I'm on all these committees and you have to educate them. They don't know what to do realistically and they keep making mistakes unless you are there to correct them and to point out the reality. It drains you, it drains you. . . . But it is satisfying because you can see you are making things better.
>
> (Woman ex-service user)

Another woman we interviewed spoke movingly in the following words:

> If they listen to us it is just so good. It makes the services better, just much better. No one has ever listened to us before. And then suddenly these posh organisations are. It brings tears to my eyes just thinking about it.

Such a positive outcome is dependent on the consultation and participation strategies in use being effective, supportive and building on strengths. How then can such outcomes be ensured? What policies are needed and how can they best be made to work? These issues will be explored in the next chapter.

Chapter 7

How to do it

Policies, sensitivities and resources to make the participation effective

In this chapter, we move on to consider the practicalities of survivor involvement. Beginning with a brief discussion of power issues in this context, we then consider consultation as part of official, legislative and policy requirements, and the need for sound and concrete policies, whatever type of participation is being considered. We then discuss some of the difficult issues that need to be part of any strategy for user involvement. These include safety, representativeness, diversity issues, and the need for resources and support. The chapter ends by opening up a discussion of what works and what does not, with a particular focus on the limited strategy of inviting individual survivors to attend policy meetings and forums on behalf of other woman, a strategy which we found in our study to be often inappropriate, upsetting and ineffective.

In general, it is of little point engaging in consultation and participation policies, as we have indicated in previous chapters, if nothing changes as a result and if the exercise remains cosmetic rather than an integrated part of policy and service delivery. However, many studies of consultative strategies with service users have found that such a tokenistic outcome is common. Consultation is carried out but there is no link between this and actual progress (Lindow and Morris, 1995). A clear issue here is who has power (see also Chapter 3), how it is operated and how much it is shared.

Power and who has it

Where agencies retain all the power and the service users being consulted have very little, it is clear that the most likely outcome is that nothing much will change if users voice their issues and concerns. Thus, there has to be a shift if effective user participation is to be possible. This can be hard to bring about, however. In general, service user involvement is widely viewed as difficult to achieve and as hampered by social exclusion and by inadequate understandings of the operation of power, as discussed in earlier sections (see, for example, Beresford and Croft, 1995; Stewart and Taylor, 1996). In fact, clarity about power issues and about who can or cannot make decisions is vital to avoid confused or muddled outcomes.

In the specific case of domestic violence, the impacts of existing power differences between service providers and service users within agencies are likely to be compounded by stark and hurtful power issues between the abuser and the woman being abused (which may, perhaps, be still continuing in post-separation harassment or through child contact). Thus, the effects can be especially reinforcing and painful. It is particularly distressing, for instance, when multi-agency forums attempt to involve survivors but do so in a way that victimises them all over again. An example would be where the woman being consulted is overlooked, not allowed to speak, or made to feel stupid during the participation process, outcomes she may have experienced countless times in abusive situations at home. Thus, the power dynamics between policy-maker and service user can mirror in an unfortunate and disturbing way those between abuser and abused. At best, of course, as discussed earlier, survivors can be empowered by a process that may contradict their previous experiences of victimisation. At worst, conversely, these negative experiences can be merely confirmed.

One woman, experienced in user participation strategies, illustrated both these outcomes in her own words. She described the power issue as follows:

> It is all about power, *all* about power, You have to understand that in a very deep way – it's not all obvious or straightforward – power takes many, often hidden, forms. Survivors don't have it. People in the agencies have to let go some of their power. And they don't want to – they just want to come to meetings and discuss it! You can struggle on as best you can but, unless they let go of some of the power – hopeless task – hopeless.

But her experiences had also led her to feel optimistic:

> Domestic violence is to do with power – so the problems with getting the agencies to share their power plays into all of this. All the power stuff can get reinforced. On the other hand, if the survivor accountability works, it is the most wonderful thing, quite amazing, and it challenges all that other stuff.

Shifting power, at least in small ways, towards domestic violence survivors, then, is what meaningful survivor involvement and accountability is all about. We move on now to look at ways of trying to do so.

Consultation with service users as part of local and central government strategy, legislation and policy

One way of trying to ensure that survivor participation is effective (though falling short of genuine accountability) and to increase the power and status of those being consulted is to use the legislative channels that have opened up in recent years in terms of formal requirements for user involvement, as we briefly discussed in previous chapters. Using such channels, survivor voices are given weight and their prominence is magnified and officially sanctioned. Such sanctioned consultation with service users, or with the general public, has now been 'mainstreamed' and is embedded in much new social policy and legislation, placing a duty of partnership and consultation on all designated authorities. Depending on the legislation or policy in question, it is required, relevant, or at least possible for strategic consultation both to focus on women who have experienced domestic violence in order to seek their views, and to include diversity of representation. (In almost all cases, of course, any consultative process will include domestic violence survivors, as both service users and professionals, but they may not have disclosed their abuse, or the consultation may be on an unrelated subject.)

Thus the setting and meeting of targets and performance indicators by professionals working with such legislation can be combined with innovatory consultation with survivors of abuse, or groups of survivors, and those who represent them. As discussed later in this chapter, over-bureaucratic and long-winded mechanisms may result in rather formal and stilted results or in the consultation losing participants. Outcomes of this type of consultation may well be rather cosmetic and, in any case, may facilitate only the most basic form of user involvement (as compared with fuller user involvement and participation leading on to agency accountability), in which those being consulted have almost no power in the process. However, where consultation which is an official part of legislation is carried out creatively with domestic violence service users, and is acted upon in practical ways, the use of such embedded and required procedures can be of some use. They may, for example, give the consultative process more authority, and ensure that agencies do not push the consultation to one side or forget to do it. At best, this type of officially required exercise may result in policy change through accepted channels defined by legislation. Where consultation is not part of required procedures in this way, there may be a tendency for agencies to overlook it or not to take it seriously. Thus, now that domestic violence policy and service development are taking place across the board, it is particularly important that required consultation procedures are used as a constructive and sensitive way of building on abused women's expressed views and wishes.

For example, through the 1998 Crime and Disorder Act, Crime and Disorder Partnerships are required to engage in extensive public consultation and, within this, are encouraged to consider domestic violence. Both of these provisions can be especially relevant and useful for women experiencing abuse. Partnerships are required to draw up Crime and Disorder Audits, in which they are expected to include the nature and profile of domestic violence in their locality. They must then consult with relevant bodies and the public in drawing up a Crime and Disorder Strategy based on the Audit. Provisions in the legislation for consultation include public meetings (usually unsuitable for discussions of domestic violence), surveys and networking. Women who have experienced domestic violence are placed in the 'hard-to-reach' category in the legislation (and, in practice, may also be 'hard to hear' for reasons explored earlier). Possible methods for reaching them that are recommended by government include the convening of (possibly disguised) public meetings in safe venues used by the hard-to-reach group in question; convening special groups; using existing forums (but for another purpose in this case); holding special conferences; and using focus groups. The Home Office also suggests that women's specialist refuge and support agencies can assist with such consultation. (See www.homeoffice.gov.uk [crime reduction].)

Similarly, Best Value is a wide-reaching and comprehensive programme to ensure high standards of service, crossing many areas of policy and provision. It requires consultation at all levels and relevant targets need to be met within Best Value performance plans and performance indicators. Within their overall plans, local authorities are required to conduct Best Value performance reviews on selected topics in terms of the four 'Cs', of which *Consult* is one. (The others are *Challenge*, *Compare* and *Compete*.) It is possible to conduct Best Value reviews on domestic violence, and the London Boroughs of Croydon and Haringey, among others, have carried out specialist exercises of this type. Extensive consultation with service users is a feature of these reviews. Domestic violence survivors and specialist domestic violence service providers have also participated in addressing the *Challenge* category. (See Office of the Deputy Prime Minister: www.odpm.gov.uk [local government].)

Supporting People, the new programme for providing housing-related services to vulnerable people, is required to establish working partnerships of local authorities, support agencies and service users. The Supporting People initiative, now the major funding source for refuge-based services, requires user consultation and aims to engage in transparent decision-making (see www.detr.gov.uk [supporting people]). There are also extensive consultation strategies within the health service, and public involvement is now an intrinsic part of NHS practice (for instance, extensive public consultation preceded the publication of the ten-year NHS Plan). Each health authority is required to produce a Health Improvement Programme (HImP), a strategic framework for improving health and reducing inequalities in health in local areas. Extensive consultation is required in the production of the HImP, with user involvement throughout the process, rather than as a one-off or 'paper' exercise. Domestic violence is clearly of relevance within HImPs and new methods of consultation are currently being developed across the country, including within health action zones. (See www.doh.gov.uk.)

There are many other partnership groupings which are required by new legislation, including local strategic partnerships within local authority areas that include voluntary sector and community representatives. The Local Government Act 2000 requires local authorities to consult with community members to prepare Community Strategies and to build the strength and capacity of the voluntary sector, which is of course the site of much independent women's support and refuge provision (see www. detr.gov.uk). Other partnerships, including Children and Young People's Strategic Partnerships involving young people and their parents or carers, require community participation. All of these complex new provisions add to previous legislation and policy that require consultation and community involvement (the 1990 NHS and Community Care Act and the production of Community Care Plans, for example). All can potentially be of use in listening to the voices of domestic violence survivors and improving domestic violence provision and services.

There can be problems, however, where high-level partnerships duplicate each other's work and when large amounts of time are spent elaborating lengthy strategies and plans of little practical impact. Difficulties can also arise if management-level interventions are imposed on otherwise grass-roots participative strategies (Barnes et al., 1999). In one locality that fed information into our study, women survivors' involvement and a 'bottom-up' domestic violence forum that had been painstakingly developed over a decade were overlooked in new partnership policy development within the local authority concerned. The forum was then replaced, with no consultation or notice, by a high-level management forum to satisfy new legislation. While the situation was finally reversed, after a time-consuming and draining struggle, it appeared for some time that the careful work of survivor consultation and the development of local policies over many years were to no avail within an over-enthusiastic and ill-informed embracing of legislation ostensibly based on partnership and user involvement. This outcome was a chilling example of organisations 'on the ground' being overlooked by over eager or messianic policy-makers and managers using 'consultation', 'partnership' and 'multi-agency' as buzz words, rather than active principles.

The need for sound policies to address sensitivities and difficulties

In general, the participation of abused women can be very significant for policy development because individual accounts may highlight issues – notably safety – that professionals may underemphasise. However, as can be seen from the foregoing discussions, consultation (let alone fuller user involvement) is a difficult thing to do well unless specific sensitivities and difficulties are recognised and addressed. For the women being consulted, these obstacles may include, as discussed earlier: safety and confidentiality issues; the impacts of poverty, of social class and of cultural imperatives and differences; the silencing and stigmatising effects of domestic violence; the impact of abuse on self-esteem; and personal difficulties in dealing with painful memories and remembered traumas.

As we have discussed, seeking service user views can in some cases result in the exploitation of the woman being consulted and in a type of 're-victimisation' – in this case, by the services concerned, rather than by the original abuser. In others, the consultation may lead nowhere or may be skilfully overlooked when the professionals do not want survivors to be part of a decision:

> It is easy for them to overlook you – even if they pretend they are not doing so! They overlook you when it is an important issue, make the 'real decisions' behind your back, call a special meeting you are not invited to – or ask you to leave at the key moment! So you have to build it one bit at a time.
>
> (Woman survivor of abuse,
> active in consultative roles)

Other service user advocacy organisations and self-organised user groups have also encountered this difficulty, and agencies in a variety of fields have a tendency to use management tactics to de-legitimise user groups when they choose to do so (Barnes *et al.*, 1999). Barnes *et al.* suggest that government injunctions to listen to user voices have had some effect in terms of improving agency attitudes. However, they point out that, as long as managers see their roles as being to 'hold the ring' between a plurality of stakeholders of whom service users are only one, and all of whom are regarded equally, it is inevitable that they will continue to attend only selectively to service user voices and will quite likely reduce them to those of 'consumers' as opposed to experts in their own lives (ibid.: 107).

In order to overcome these various difficulties, there is an indisputable need for the use of an agreed and sensitive procedure or mechanism for consultation with abused women, which agencies are obliged to follow and which is accepted as an automatic part of policy. The integration of such procedures into agency operation is vital, rather than just 'hoping it will happen'. Nevertheless, we identified examples in our research of inter-agency forums, in particular, adopting the latter approach, especially where there was a refuge involved that might, just by its presence, be assumed by others to ensure that consultation had happened when it had never in reality been mooted as a possibility.

Conversely, while an agreed procedure for any participation process is essential, we also found that an overly bureaucratic approach and too much procedure could actually kill it off. Rather, simple and clear steps were required. To be meaningful and effective, the findings of many other service user movements were echoed in this study in that consultation needs several elements (see Department of Health 1996a, 1996b). These include:

- the actual consultation and creative, sensitive ways to carry it out, cognisant of equality and diversity issues;
- a mechanism for converting the result of the consultation into real action and policy change;
- a mechanism for reviewing this, for making sure it happens and for keeping those consulted apprised of outcomes.

Procedures to govern each of these three vital components of effective user involvement are essential for domestic violence services. These may include agreed, specific protocols for multi-agency forums or individual agencies on user participation and on developing service standards to meet the demands expressed (see also Chapter 10). Ideally, women survivors can participate in the design and planning of policies and protocols, or can set up and control mechanisms for involvement and accountability themselves, although this is rarely achieved at present. Self-activity and user control are a long way down the line in most cases, where typically at present only basic consultation has been attempted.

Moreover, many organisations in the domestic violence field, as in others, consult and then fail to do anything with the results. The second and third parts of the process outlined above get overlooked, sometimes because those conducting the consultation run out of steam to take it further or don't have the power to do so. This outcome is not only dismissive of those being consulted, but could also be said to be 'setting domestic violence survivors up to fail'. As we have consistently emphasised, there is also a clear differ-ence between simple consultation, on the one hand, and real involvement or accountability, on the other, in which survivors can make or contribute to decisions and have some actual power in the organisation.

There have been attempts in several other user groups to raise issues of genuine accountability. Mental health service users, for example, have attempted to hold service purchasers and providers accountable:

'To put them in the hot seat if you like', in order to get them to explain directly to users why they are not providing the service people want.

(Barnes *et al.*, 1999: 93)

Members of the British Council of Disabled People, the longest established coalition in the country, have the increased accountability of services to such users as a priority aim. They point out that organisations are not used to being answerable to service users or having to respond to awkward questions (ibid.: 99). It is a difficult struggle for user groups to get them to do so, not only within the fields of disability and mental health, but also in the domestic violence field.

We need, then, to begin perhaps with consultation strategies, as long as they are meaningful ones, but always to attempt to engage in – and to move on to – fuller participatory strategies which lead towards true accountability of agencies to their users. In embarking on this challenging road, agencies and inter-agency forums wishing to develop effective user participation strategies in respect of women experiencing domestic violence, and to avoid some of the outcomes referred to above, may wish, as a first step, to make use of the basic checklist in Box 7.1 to assess both their position and possible ways of improving it. The list can be used to develop participation mechanisms further in different agencies and inter-agency forums. Sound policies which address the local situation and which are simple to understand, non-bureaucratic and transparent can then be evolved, developed and funded. Such policies may change and develop over time as conditions change. Thus, the endeavour of survivor participation needs to be an ongoing process which, rather than coming to completion, needs constant development and refining in a sensitive way.

Whatever the participation or consultation procedure that is put in place, all the views expressed need to be heeded. A challenging and somewhat thorny matter concerns what happens when survivors being consulted express different views to their representatives or to those of advocacy and support agencies and feminist activists. What is to be done if 'they' – abused women – do not say what 'we' – the feminists – want them to? While this can be a painful and difficult process, it may be the case that robust differences of view can lead to the development of more rounded policy over time, and that those with the most recent experience of abuse can challenge potential complacency in others who may believe that their hard work and political analysis have solved problems which, in fact, still remain.

Safety, representativeness and diversity

Key issues to be addressed in any attempt to involve abuse survivors in policy or service development include the need for their safety and

Box 7.1   Basic initial checklist

- Is your agency already conducting service user consultation with abused women?
- Is this consultation resulting in changes in policy and service provision?
- Are any resultant changes reviewed regularly with feedback to those consulted?
- Do women survivors have any wider influence on your policy-making?
- Do women survivors have any real power to make decisions or to contribute directly to policy-making in your agency or project?

- Does your local inter-agency domestic violence forum have mechanisms in place for seeking the views of women service users on its work across the locality?
- Are these mechanisms being used and do they work? How do you know that they work?

- Is there a women's refuge organisation, outreach or other specialist domestic violence service in your area? If so, is your agency able to liaise with it?
- Are any refuge or outreach organisations in a position to feed in, or to act as a conduit for, the views of abused women using services to agencies or the forum?

- In your local area, to what extent can women service users contribute to:
    - Inter-agency domestic violence forums or local inter-agency strategy groups?
    - Crime and Disorder Partnerships and other partnership groups?
    - Local health trusts?
    - The police and criminal justice agencies?
    - Local authorities and their departments, e.g. social services, education and housing?
    - Refuge and support organisations or other women's advocacy projects?
    - General service and policy development on a single or multi-agency basis?
    - Any local public education and awareness-raising initiatives?
- Are there simple changes by which this could be improved?
- What are the potential barriers to change?
- What exists already that could be positively built on?

confidentiality to be paramount at all times, an essential requirement that can work against transparent consultation processes. Safe methods of contacting abused women, in particular, must be conducted with great care. Further, both venues used and transport there and back need to be safe, anonymous and secure. If the involvement in policy-making of women who have experienced violence leads to their further abuse and to safety issues being overlooked, then clearly bad, dangerous or even disastrous practice has taken place. These matters are of the utmost importance and should override all other considerations.

Other contentious issues to be considered include the accountability of those being consulted. Are they in fact answerable to anyone and, if so, to whom? Commonly accepted democratic structures that ensure representativeness are not applicable, and highly organised accountable groups may be impossible to establish in this area of work. This issue is typically raised against service user groups and, as we suggested in Chapter 3, can become a barrier to empowerment. Lack of representativeness is frequently used by agencies and policy-makers as a reason – even an excuse – for not taking user participation seriously. In the domestic violence field, the difficulty can be magnified by issues of confidentiality and on occasion the need for security and an element of secrecy.

Domestic violence service users clearly only represent themselves unless they are present as members of a survivors' group. But, bearing in mind the points made above and in Chapter 3, this may or may not matter. Their contributions are likely to be less worthwhile:

> It's a representative issue. It's hard if survivors are told they don't represent anyone so 'are not valid'. Women representing themselves. The survivors on the forum felt they weren't accepted, weren't valid. That's how they were made to feel. But, what survivors say is crucial to inform policy. The answer to 'how are they representative?': 'It doesn't matter. They are representing themselves – this is enough in itself'. Don't expect survivors to represent anyone except themselves but that is valuable, it's enough.
>
> (Worker in an empowerment project who
> had facilitated a survivors' forum)

Representativeness, though, cannot be abandoned altogether. To do so would open the field to skewed responses where, for example, only survivors who were personally known to the workers as holding positive views might be consulted about services in an agency. However, it can never be perfectly achieved either. Our study findings led to the recommendation that policy-makers engaging in user participation and consultation exercises should attempt to ensure as democratic a structure as possible, learning from other service user consultations in process, but taking on board the specific sensitivities and traumas of domestic violence. One partial solution is to involve existing support or self-help organisations of survivors, which can give a distilled and collaborative view while also offering support to members. Thus, where support groups and survivors within advocacy projects can be consulted or involved in other ways, the process may be more sympathetic and the outcomes more representative than in situations where isolated individuals are involved. But, in either case, the voices still plug a gap that professionals can never fill. Users of services can always make specific comments on the service they have received personally and, if policy-makers feel there has been some attempt at representation, they are more likely to be responsive and to view the consultation positively.

There is a further issue of diversity within representation. We now recognise that domestic violence is astoundingly common, probably affecting more than one in four women across a lifetime (Stanko et al., 1998). Women of all backgrounds, social classes, ethnicities, cultures, sexualities, nationalities and degrees of disability can experience it (Davies, 1994; Hague and Malos, 1998). In such a context, complete representativeness can become meaningless. An issue of considerable importance and complexity, then, becomes how to address equality and diversity within survivor representation. Thus, when developing and formalising new policy and practice on domestic violence, it is essential to seek a variety of views from an inclusive sample of abused women (including for example, women from minority communities, disabled women and so on). It is also of importance to seek views from a wide range of individuals, groups and organisations, including survivors, clearly, but also including advocacy organisations, and other agencies as relevant.

Some agencies, however, may be tempted to rely on consultation with a very few survivors who may not represent a sufficiently comprehensive view of the diverse needs of women who experience domestic abuse. For example, consulting only with refuge residents may not reveal the problems facing those in other forms of temporary accommodation. When policy-makers are desperate to set up, or to be seen to set up, consultation strategies, it can be tempting to involve whoever can be found. This may mean, for example, that only white women participate, even in multiracial localities, or that disabled people are excluded, possibly because it is too troublesome to locate relevant individuals or groups or to facilitate communication for those with visual or hearing impairments. There is a clear need to ensure that domestic violence survivors participating are drawn from all sections of the community.

Formal attempts at quotas to represent different communities do not seem to work well and lead to over-prescriptive responses on occasion, but less formal approaches are possible. Specialist consultation with specific minority groups can be very helpful in feeding into broader strategies.

For instance, focused discussions with disabled women's groups, or with black women and children, may be able to tap into specific needs and to raise voices which often go unheard. In one example, the Community Safety Unit of the Metropolitan Police in the London Borough of Brent has set up a series of consultation meetings with the long-standing Asian Women's Resource Centre, including with survivors of violence, to develop ways of reaching Asian women suffering abuse and of combating the assumed under-reporting of domestic violence in their communities (Hague, 2002). These issues are re-examined in terms of specific, practical methods in the chapters that follow.

It is work after all: resources and support

What works in developing participative and consultative mechanisms in the field of domestic violence is a complex matter, as discussed earlier. Effective processes are likely to be those that deal in a deliberate and careful manner with all the issues outlined above and that revise and revisit them regularly. All of this takes time and energy for both workers and service users. One survivor we interviewed told us that 'you can't do it in a hurry – it takes a while, plus input and resources, but it can be done'. This woman went on to explain some of the difficulties in this endeavour:

> There is a gap between policies and what is happening on the ground. It is wonderful to empower women but not to set them up to fail. We need more support and resources to avoid this. Usually it's hypocrisy, 'We all listen to survivors.' People say this but they don't really mean it. Then it raises hopes but no one is saying, 'We will support them to do this.' No one is saying, 'We will take account of what we hear.' So it can all just be naivety. Pretence. It's no good setting it up not to work. Or setting it up in order to then ignore it. It needs to be resourced – it's not a cheap thing and it's not easy either.
>
> (Survivor active in consultation processes)

Thus, consultation and user participation cannot be done on the cheap. To be effective, they also need to be embedded in policy development. For this to happen, they must be an official and accepted part of budgets, automatically written in and expected in all grant applications and budgetary plans. Barnes et al. (1999) emphasise that, in general, policy-makers who are genuinely committed to involving service user groups in the design, planning and delivery of services need to encourage and financially support not only their own consultation processes, but also, in the words of these authors, the self-organisation of users without their being 'captured by or incorporated into management' (ibid.: 107). The key issues here are independence of operation and financial support. Groups of service users do not often have access to their own resources and may be left wide open to being used by local authorities and other agencies without compensation.

In order to avoid the risk of exploiting abused women, our study identified a whole raft of issues around making the 'giving' two-way, so that women involved also 'receive'. Such concerns are clearly recognised and are the subject of detailed recommendations among other service user groups and in Department of Health guidance (see Lindow, 1994; Department of Health, 1996a, 1996b). They include the need for resources, compensation of various kinds, training and support, if service users are to be enabled to participate effectively.

In the domestic violence field, then, as in others where service user voices are raised, user participation needs to be sensitive to a complexity of resource issues. Taking part in consultative and participative structures is clearly work for those being consulted, just as it is for the professionals involved. In our study we found that it is quite important to take on board the reality of this statement, but that many agencies do not do so. We need to ask ourselves why service providers who participate in consultation are funded and supported, while abused women are expected to participate in their spare time and out of kindness, goodwill or personal commitment.

In general, there is an uncomfortable disjuncture where salaried professionals depend on the unpaid work of service users who have experienced abuse. It is essential that women who have experienced domestic violence and who offer their services in this way should be offered expenses, at the very least, together with transport to and from any meetings and childcare, either directly provided or reimbursed. These are the basics that need to be in place, come what may, as fundamental core good practice. Better still, proper payment for the work conducted needs to be considered and provided wherever possible, so that participants are recompensed for their labour and effort. Where money is available this is clearly best practice, although few inter-agency forums or agencies have such resources readily to hand and care is required to ensure that payments do not put users' benefits at risk.

In fact, this is a new issue in respect to domestic violence services, and the debate about payment is only just beginning. Some domestic violence survivors' groups feel that, while payment is always a positive option, it is not necessarily the only way forward, claiming that women participants need to gain something from their participation, but that this can be payment in kind or in increased self-confidence and self-esteem. Other forms of reciprocity can include outings, talks or training courses (although, arguably, these should be available to all women). These may be able to be funded through budgets that do not allow for direct payment of participants. What is important is that women engaging in consultation or participation mechanisms are not 'used', but how they are recompensed may vary according to circumstances and the needs of the women concerned.

Human and financial resources are also needed in other ways. The provision of interpreting and translation facilities is vital to reach women whose first language is not English, although care needs to be taken over confidentiality and the selection of appropriate and sympathetic interpreters from relevant communities. They should certainly never be the woman's children and they need to work to professional standards to ensure accuracy and confidentiality. Any meetings held need to be sited in sympathetic venues, which are also safe and secure for women who have experienced violence to attend in a way that does not mark them out for attention and that facilitates a ready alibi if one is required. Venues need to be accessible and safe in all ways. This may mean, for example, that attention needs to be paid to how generally safe the locality around the venue is for women and whether it is known as a racist area. All meetings need to be conducted with respectful attention to women's needs, to cultural differences and to possible discrimination. Thus, cultural sensitivity and awareness of all equality issues need to form an integral part of consultation mechanisms, and to include provision for disabled women. The latter is likely to include ensuring there is good disabled access to venues, as well as the provision of appropriate transport and the availability of any necessary documents in large print or on tape, with sign language interpreting available on request, all of which have resource implications.

Very probably, agency workers in the field are offered in-service support and training. The question then needs to be asked as to why women service users being consulted or contributing to the work of agencies in other ways usually are not. User involvement as part of policy development can be extremely problematic and demanding for domestic violence survivors, and to engage in it without extra training and help can be a negative experience for the women concerned and damaging, or at least ineffective, all round. Thus, abused women may need initial induction and training, support and, possibly, consultancy of their own. This is likely to be particularly the case if they have formed an ongoing group. Training can assist members of the group to act as effective representatives, to develop their skills and to overcome management obstacles to user involvement. Workers in Women's Aid who were consulted during our study recommended that users and ex-users participating in management committees or undertaking volunteer work in refuges could be offered mentoring or 'buddying' services and provided with support and training to overcome the complexities and difficulties of switching from a user role to a provider one. Other agencies could also benefit from this advice.

To take on all of these issues clearly needs resource input. Again, successful user participation and consultation is something that cannot be done with tiny amounts of money cobbled together at the last minute, as is so often the case in practice. They must be adequately costed into the budget. In fact, our study found that resource shortage is the most likely reason for participation strategies to fail. Which groups are supported financially can also be an issue. Funding for consultative groups that are specially created for the purpose by statutory agencies may be attracted by making coherent arguments for their importance in funding applications. They can then be built into agency strategic and operational imperatives so that they can be justified in all future budgets. While this can be a positive way forward, the independence of such groups may be compromised in some ways and they may be manipulated on occasion by powerful organisations or professionals. Self-organised user groups, on the other hand, are likely to be more independent but are known to be chronically unstable in terms of funding (Barnes *et al.*, 1999: 107), which makes them difficult to maintain in the long term. Thus, resourcing for user groups of all types is important in order to facilitate user involvement, and should not be limited to certain types of intervention, given the range of possible initiatives and variation. Further, the resources need to be adequate to the task. A very small amount of money granted to user consultation can be problematic to administer and may take more time to justify and account for than it 'buys'. The granting of such monies may make agencies look good in terms of appearing to take on the issue, and feel good in terms of their own committedness to an innovative cause, but may make no difference in reality.

To reiterate, then – for user participation to be an effective, viable and integrated part of service delivery, it needs to be taken seriously and properly resourced as an automatic part of funding strategy and of service and policy development, built into budgets and regarded as an essential part of the policy process. Independent advocacy groups can play a particularly valuable role and require more generalised support with finance. Overall, the resources provided need to be adequate to the task if effective outcomes are to be achieved.

The Westminster Domestic Violence Forum, which is discussed in Chapter 8, is a model of good practice in this respect. Their survivors' forum, which works alongside the forum as a whole, was integrated into the operation from the very beginning, rather than being something which was thought about and added on later. The original budget of the forum, though small, had an item built into it for the financial support of consultation with women using services. Thus, the involvement of women survivors was an integral, funded part of the project from the start and, ever since, has been automatically accepted by all participants.

What works and what does not: individual survivors attending meetings

As we have noted, our research found that there is no one way of consulting and involving domestic violence survivors. What evolves in a locality will clearly depend on local conditions and sometimes on local personalities. The various innovative methods and strategies currently in use will be discussed in the ensuing chapters (Chapters 8, 9 and 10).

However, the most common method that has been tried by inter-agency forums and other projects involves service users attending policy or inter-agency forum meetings in person. In this approach, one or two survivors participate in forum meetings to put the 'survivor view'. This can be useful for the professionals present to anchor and illuminate discussions, but there are many difficulties associated with it. Agencies may want the right to meet together on their own, at least sometimes, to strategise and to support each other, given how difficult their task is in overcoming the obstacles to joint working, in putting in place effective interventions and in dealing with the distressing nature of the subject itself. Thus, it may not always be appropriate to have service users or ex-users attending forum meetings. From the survivors' point of view, individuals placed in this situation may be overwhelmed or damaged by the experience, although this can be ameliorated if substantial and careful support is provided.

Our study found that, in reality, this individualised approach to representation rarely works (unless remarkable personalities are involved), especially if everyone else at the meeting attended is representing an agency and may be quite senior within it, with access to decision-making. If women users participating in policy meetings are representing a women's project or support group, and therefore have a function as representatives of a wider organisation in common with the other professional participants, this may work better. In general, though, this type of consultation is a difficult thing to achieve. Various agencies with whom we talked had tried to make it work but said that women did not wish to attend, as the agency worker quoted here explains:

> We set up all the procedures and tried to make it comfortable for women to come but, when they did, they didn't like it and then, after that, no one came. So then we tried to set up separate meetings but women did not want to come to those, either, after we'd spent a long time organising it. We were disappointed but we will have to think of something else.

Even where women can be supported to attend and wish to do so, the difficulties can be almost insurmountable, especially when the professionals all have more education and more knowledge about their agencies, about service provision and about agency and meeting culture than the service users or ex-users are likely to have. One woman survivor whom we interviewed had this to say:

It's hard for survivors to attend forum meetings where everyone else is a professional, however welcoming they try to be. You still feel small and as though you shouldn't be there when they are all professionals. It's probably best to consult survivors in other ways.

Another said:

Having women on the committees and doing survivor accountability – yes, good idea but only if the women are confident enough. But they can be cosmetic. ... In fact, the survivors on the committee have no power at all. But, if there is a women's group, rather than being on your own, that is better – you would not be so isolated but would be representing the group.

It can be seen from these quotes that survivors' voices are often muted by the official milieu. At worst, abused women who are attending may be viewed voyeuristically by the professionals and may be placed, even without anyone meaning this to happen, in the category of being a 'specimen'. This possibility is likely to be extremely upsetting for the individual survivors involved. Service users attending meetings in this way are, almost by definition, heavily outnumbered and may also feel overwhelmed by management and agency procedure, confidence and formalities. Such experiences are often distressing and inappropriate for the individuals involved (although involvement of service users in this way has been successful on some occasions). Survivors interviewed in our study reported feeling silenced and patronised or, on occasion, subject to potentially racist or discriminatory responses from agency workers, even where the agencies or forums concerned were trying hard to avoid these outcomes.

Other service users who were interviewed reported constant amazement at the 'talking shop' nature of many official meetings and the apparent waste of time involved. One woman put this view as follows:

They are better than they were, much better. But there is so much talk – conferences, forums, publications, fanfare – but what's changed? Has it really changed? Not really.

She continued succinctly:

They say in their fancy suits that they are doing all these things at their meetings – the 'talk culture' – always the 'talk culture' – but for women it's not much different, is it?

Policy-making may be unnecessarily time-consuming, boring and tedious, and there are also issues to be considered in relation to the use of language and of alienating 'meeting culture' working practices. All of these matters necessitate the provision of ongoing support and training for abused women involved in this work. An interviewee pointed out:

> Language, you know, 'middle-class meeting language'. Sometimes it helps, it is shorthand for something. But usually it is actually unnec-essary – alienating and intimidating.

Once again, these issues are compounded for ethnic minority women. In the following quote from a black woman survivor and project worker, domestic violence forums, strategies and policy-making are tersely char-acterised by three 'Bs':

> Bureaucratic . . . big . . . no black people.

In conclusion: a positive experiment

The Westminster Domestic Violence Forum is discussed in the next chapter and works alongside a survivors' group called the Phoenix Group. This group has been meeting for some years and recently came to a point where the members considered asking to attend the forum meetings directly. The facilitator discussed this possibility with all concerned, including asking the main forum members, not only what they thought about the proposal, but also what they felt about it. The decision by all concerned in this case was that the participation of members of the Phoenix Group in the full forum was not the best use of everyone's resources (although it could be so in the future). It was decided that it would be more effective if they worked as members of individual sub-groups of the forum to participate in and contribute to specific pieces of work in order to make inputs that led to real changes.

Women from the Phoenix Group now attend the Prevention Strategy Sub-group which has developed a schools domestic violence prevention pack, and they spoke at the launch of this pack. The women also attend the Training Sub-group and participated in the development of a training pack and the making of a video. They are currently in the process of making a further video with the police to be used to train frontline police officers on domestic violence. Through being involved in these constructive projects, the Phoenix Group members have been able to see directly that they have an active and practical role to play in these sub-groups and can contribute in a real way. Their contributions have led to the groups concerned achieving more than they otherwise would have done. All involved agreed that the women from the Phoenix Group were there with a function and had a real role, rather than being labelled as users or being present merely as tokens. The interaction of agency representatives and women from the group has been particularly creative for everyone involved. Some of the women group members said:

> We've been respected at the meetings we've attended of the Forum sub-groups . . . we are contributing with our experienced voices to the Forum's work.

Both the Phoenix Group and the main Forum are facilitated particularly sensitively, even uniquely, and this facilitation and support has undoubtedly helped to achieve such positive outcomes. Nevertheless, other domestic violence forums may be able to learn from these experiences.

In conclusion, our study found that consultation and the involvement of abused women can be an emotionally powerful and passionate process for all concerned, including the policy-makers themselves. It is an essential component of policy and practice in order to keep government, local authority, police and other policy developments on track, and to make services effective and geared towards women and children's real needs. It is not an 'optional extra'.

A member of an inter-agency forum that had managed to be successful in incorporating survivor representatives had this to say:

> They [the survivor representatives] are there as a right and have equal say with anyone else. They can raise any issues and will always be listened to. For example, we took up the anti-discrimination and 'no men' policies from survivors' comments and the need for a helpline came from women and is being actually done now.

A survivor involved with a different forum told us that:

> Women should be involved so agencies can be more effective. So women who've had all their power taken away can have a voice. Be part of the decision-making process on some level. Not necessarily by attending formal meetings, though. . . . But, when they do it, it results in safer services. Policies that are being agreed are checked on by survivors.

In summary, the involvement of abused women is clearly a demanding and sensitive issue to address, although it is also an extremely rewarding and exciting one, especially when it works well. It needs to be carried out, not just as a formality, but according to an agreed procedure which has a real effect and which leads to policy change and action. Our study found that few agencies and professionals are attempting it at the moment (even at the most basic level of consultation), and the individual and collective empowerment of abused women that it could herald remains principally confined to the women's activist movement. There is a clear need for inter-agency forums and agencies in the statutory sector to pay attention to the matter, and to put in place effective policies that are properly resourced in a sensitive and creative way. Consultation and participation are work, after all, and need to be accompanied by finances, expenses, training and support. There is no one easy answer, but seeking the views of domestic violence survivors does offer a challenging and rewarding way ahead.

Chapter 8

Practical ways forward and innovation, including domestic violence survivors' forums

> The humanness of trying it is what is so important and is often overlooked by boring procedures and doing it because you feel you have to, not because you are committed to it. You need the humanity of it. You need to do it on a deep 'felt and lived' level as human beings, as equals in the endeavour. Survivor accountability is a real human thing and it touches all levels. What we have learned from trying to do it here is that the people who are doing it need great commitment and humanity and depth.
>
> (Agency worker)

'You need the humanity of it.' This powerful quote is from an agency employee working with groups of domestic violence survivors to develop ways of raising their voices and feeding their views into the policy-making process. In previous chapters, we discussed the complex general issues involved in engaging in survivor participation and consultation within domestic violence projects. In the next three chapters, we move on to discuss some of the innovative methods that are currently being tried. While inter-agency domestic violence forums and specialist projects generally appear at present to have little expertise in how to go about such consultation, there are a few pioneers who are experimenting with new and exciting ways forward from which we could all perhaps learn.

An example: Hammersmith Standing Together against Domestic Violence

The Hammersmith Standing Together project has developed an innovative multi-agency response to domestic violence, modelled, broadly speaking, on the Domestic Abuse Intervention Project in Duluth, Minnesota. One of its founding principles is 'putting the survivor at the centre of the change process' (Standing Together, 2002: 9). Standing Together believes in the empowerment of women and that:

where agencies plan change, however well-intentioned, without the involvement of people with current, first-hand knowledge of the issues, there is a serious risk that the safety of women and children will be diminished rather then increased.

(ibid.: 9)

The project carried out a detailed consultation with domestic violence survivors in 2001–2, being repeated in 2003, and conducted by a consultant and assistant experienced in such work. An important innovation which might be of help to others was the drawing up of a protocol on how the whole exercise would be carried out. The protocol committed the organisation to working in respectful and supportive ways, and in which the safety of the women taking part was paramount. This was agreed with all the relevant agencies and was used to govern the process in a transparent and clear way, with detailed plans drawn up for each consultation meeting.

An attempt was made to involve as wide a range of survivors as possible and an additional consultation with black and minority ethnic women was carried out by a partner agency. Thus, the exercise as a whole reflected ethnic and other types of diversity in the community. Women were contacted by letter through the local survivors' agencies which had been involved in planning the work. Each woman was invited directly by an agency she knew, which created a sense of safety and involvement from the beginning. Meetings were then convened for those interested in taking part. The venue was carefully selected in a non-conspicuous location with a warm and welcoming atmosphere and a crèche.

Standing Together staff assisted in drawing up questions and issues to be consulted on at each meeting in order to provide a framework, but participants were also able to influence or change the process proactively. Ground rules were established by the women participants and included that each woman could choose how much or how little she wanted to say about herself. The meetings took place over several months and detailed reports were made on each. The aim was to work towards the establishment of an ongoing focus group for future consultations.

A crucial element in the success of this consultation was that sufficient resources were allocated to carry it out properly. Travel costs, childcare, refreshments and gift vouchers for each woman were provided, and some of the women were very moved to receive the latter. The employment of an external consultant who was completely outside the project assisted in facilitating objectivity, and women were enabled to speak freely about their experiences of agencies, even where this resulted in the expression of negative views. This type of distancing can be vital to ensure an accurate response.

The consultant used had extensive experience of domestic violence work, so was able to facilitate in a sensitive and supportive way, cognisant of the realities of experiencing abuse and of the need for the women to feel involved in, and committed to, the process. The result was the establishing of warm relationships between the women themselves so that they were able to 'own' and to feel invested in the consultation. The creation of the women's own 'space' to consider the issues in question undoubtedly facilitated the process and could be seen as an essential component if consultation is to be effective.

Another important element in the consultation was having a facilitator and an assistant (from different ethnic and cultural heritages), working together to complement each other and to provide support. The expression of emotions was not viewed negatively but was seen as part of the process. In this context, the fact that there were two people available meant that more intense support could be offered to individuals when required. They also modelled a respectful working relationship and the process was moving for all concerned. The facilitators stated that they felt honoured to be part of the consultation, and both they and the participants ended up changed by the experience. This project could provide a model of good practice and has been documented for others to use (Standing Together, 2002). An interesting reflection upon this successful endeavour is that 'consultation' is seen in the user involvement literature (as we discussed in Part 1) as falling at the least emancipatory end of a continuum of partic-ipation, yet it can be highly important and empowering if well conducted and thoroughgoing (perhaps a reflection on how seldom it tends to happen). This particular exercise took place in a specialist project, Standing Together. It would be good to see statutory agencies following suit, and all agencies building on this foundation to move on and involve users in other ways.

Innovatory methods now being tried

Thus, survivor involvement within domestic violence work is perfectly possible as long as it is thought about carefully, built into funding, and developed with sincerity and commitment. Sometimes, according to our interviewees, it is important to realise that it is nothing to be scared of. Rather, the important thing is to give user involvement a try in the domestic violence field, rather than being frightened of rocking the boat or of what might happen as a result. Our informants emphasised that it does need careful planning and operation, but it can be done. The woman quoted at the beginning of this chapter, who has a great deal of experience of working on survivor accountability, referred to the humanness of the endeavour, and it is perhaps vital not to lose sight of this under a welter of procedures. This remains the case even though the current emphasis on explicit consul-tative structures with users, which is part of most new policy and legislation, can be a key tool, as discussed in the last chapter.

The participation methods presently being tried in various parts of the country are listed in Box 8.1, and include survivors' forums or advisory groups, women's focus groups and the active involvement of local women's organisations, notably Women's Aid, to represent abused women's voices and to act as a conduit for information exchange. Special initiatives may also be put into place on a one-off basis and many agencies use established, but perhaps rather arid (non-participative) mechanisms such as exit questionnaires and user surveys. Liaison with activist groups is also a vital component of any consultation strategy, and political and feminist community theatre, art and poetry all have their part to play in raising the voices of abused women. Campaigns and activism have always involved grassroots projects and domestic violence survivors themselves. The anchor has traditionally been the social movement of women for liberation and justice and it continues to be so, as discussed throughout this book. In the next three chapters, we will discuss in turn each of these participation methods in order to offer ideas for the future. We will also attempt to consider where these methods fall more into the 'consultation' end of the spectrum, where they include wider involvement and participation, and where they have the potential to devolve real power to service users and to move towards the accountability of services and policies to domestic violence survivors.

Box 8.1   New and innovative practice in consultation with abused women

- Domestic violence survivors' forums or advisory groups.
- Active involvement of women's organisations, Women's Aid, and other women's projects to represent abused women's voices and to act as a conduit for information exchange.
- General liaison with agencies representing abused women, e.g. women's support groups, campaigns and refuge organisations.
- Political and community theatre and arts.
- Women's focus groups.
- Specific individual mechanisms, e.g. one-off meetings between abused women and senior managers.
- Questionnaires, surveys and research projects on service user views.
- Internet consultation.
- Regular feedback and consultation slots at, for example, domestic violence forum meetings, together with protocols for acting on them.
- Survivors and ex-service users taking roles as managers, workers and volunteers.

Domestic violence survivors' forums or advisory groups

In the good practice example of the Hammersmith Standing Together project which was described in the preceding pages, one of the aims was to establish a consultative group to look at the practice of the project and of its member agencies which would meet several times. In a few cases throughout the country, groups of this nature which are ongoing have been established over a longer period to provide a structured and sensitive mechanism for survivors, including service users, to be involved in policy development and multi-agency work.

Domestic violence survivors' forums or advisory groups consisting of abused women have been established, for example, to work together with, and alongside, some local inter-agency forums. These groups are often also support groups, and can offer an inspirational and moving way forward in which policy-makers begin to be directly accountable to abused women service users. In some cases, existing support groups may set aside time, once a month or so, to look at and comment on the work of the main inter-agency domestic violence forum in the area, as one part of their interaction, alongside their support function. In other cases, the group may only meet occasionally and may have been specifically convened to make comments on abused women's needs, on what services are required, on new service and policy initiatives and on progress in combatting domestic violence in the locality in question.

Working with survivors' forums can be a very effective consultation strategy for inter-agency forums and policy-makers in that there is an existing mechanism for accessing women's views in a transparent way which can be reviewed to make sure the consultative process happens. But survivors' forums of this type also have the potential to develop beyond consultation to involve service users and ex-users more fully in the policy process. At their best, they can become accountability committees that can advise on and monitor service development and have a deciding word on policy.

Currently, there are a few of these groups in different local authorities around the country and they are usually actively facilitated by an employee. One of the first pioneers of this approach was in the London Borough of Croydon, which ran a survivors' forum for several years until membership dropped off and the forum was brought to an end. In the study on which this book is based, we learned as much as we could about the Croydon initiative, which was flourishing at the beginning of the study but came to an end in 1999. Although ending prematurely, this forum was a pioneer of its type and a brave step into the unknown for all involved.

Croydon Domestic Violence Survivors' Forum

In the London Borough of Croydon, the domestic violence forum is one of the Borough's Joint Planning Teams, all of which are required to engage in user consultation. The Domestic Violence Survivors' Forum (DVSF) was formed as part of this requirement and was originally set up with a great deal of community support and with professional help. A sizeable number of women were involved and the project was professionally facilitated, as one of four separate community empowerment projects constituting the joint-funded Croydon Empowerment Project. Members of the group attended the Domestic Violence Joint Planning Team meetings, which was a difficult experience (as discussed in the last chapter), despite the efforts of agency representatives on the forum to be as welcoming as possible. In general, though, running a domestic violence survivors' forum was outside the working practices and experience of both the statutory and voluntary sectors in the locality at the time that it commenced and considerable learning took place.

The DVSF developed well and engaged in much useful work as a robust force for change and accountability. The women met enthusiastically and made unique contributions to combatting domestic violence in the area, with help both from the facilitator and also from the London Borough of Croydon Equalities Unit and Croydon Welcare. The Survivors' Forum began to attract interest from outside the borough, and papers and reports were written about it to give others inspiration to perhaps try something similar in their own local authorities. It was later granted a small amount of money to employ workers to action the project. However, this led to complications in regards to the need for procedures, committees, budgets and so on, even though the amount of money was negligible in wider terms and was certainly not enough to do the job effectively and comprehensively. Two survivors shared the work, which meant that each was working for only a few hours per week. These employees did the best they could with very limited time and money. Later, some energy which would have been devoted to the DVSF was diverted into the formation of the very successful Croydon One Stop Project which is discussed in Chapter 10. However, the facilitator continued to put much energy and personal resources into the project, probably beyond the call of duty.

Towards the end, women survivors requested advice sessions and the two workers started running these. However, such sessions did not fulfil the brief of survivor accountability required for the receipt of funding and the project came to an end. In an unrelated development, the funding for the Empowerment Project was cut at about the same time, demonstrating the vulnerability of such projects to changes in funding regimes unless they are firmly embedded in procedure and in the strategic commitments of the local authority or the relevant partnership or agency concerned.

The DVSF had various successes, including input into the formation of community-focused projects, support for legal representation for abused women and the provision of evidence that there was a need in the area both for advocacy for abused women and children and for a layer of support that was not professional. Most of these ideas have since been actioned in Croydon. Thus, the experiment worked well for some time and has certainly acted as a catalyst for other developments, although some interviewees felt that there were problems throughout, particularly around racial and personal differences.

In our study, we concluded that the very small amount of money granted was part of the problem. The project was almost 'set up to fail'. There was not enough money to run it properly or to keep it going in the long term, yet its existence caused bureaucratic problems. The lack of payment for members (who at this point were putting in a large amount of time on the DVSF) was another problematic factor. It can be assumed that no one else involved with the domestic violence forum or other Joint Planning Teams was likely to be doing it in their spare time for no pay.

It could be argued that the DVSF only reached certain types of survivors (those motivated to go to meetings, for example). However, it is the agency's responsibility to conduct survivor consultation successfully, not the survivors'. Thus, there needs to be something 'in it' for the women as well as for the agency. Meetings can become boring after a while, and this was the experience in Croydon. To keep such a forum going, there can be a continual need for fresh members to attend to prevent the group becoming stagnant or turned in on itself. The need to replenish the membership of user groups in general has been widely recognised (see Barnes *et al.*, 1999). Some women who moved on from the work obtained paid employment in the field, yet their previous involvement was sometimes viewed as a conflict of interest, rather than a positive enhancement of their skills. This, again, constitutes a challenge to professional agencies to accord survivors greater respect and recognition.

Ongoing groups of survivors sometimes encounter internal problems, partly due to the traumatic past that members are likely to have experienced and the difficulties of keeping any group going in the long term. After a considerable period of success, such difficulties developed to some extent in the DVSF. The lack of resources for support, training and confidence-building in the group were key factors, even though the facilitator tried hard to achieve successful outcomes. While she was herself a very skilled groupworker, she faced an almost impossible task, given the fact that she had four completely different and unrelated projects to 'empower'.

As noted in Chapter 7, local circumstances and the personalities of group members are of key importance, and this was the case in Croydon. The DVSF was an experiment in an untried area, and there were no guidelines or previous examples of similar work on which to draw. Other local authorities have more recently taken on similar work and have now gone further with it. However, at the time when the DVSF was functioning, it was at the very forefront of developments in this area of work and was in a rather isolated position. Thus the project and the local authority are to be congratulated on giving it a try. Lone initiators of new policy developments always, of course, face a difficult and potentially lonely task.

The Phoenix Group

Current examples of survivors' forums include the Phoenix Group in the City of Westminster and Voice for Change in Liverpool, both of which are currently working successfully and are able to influence policy development and the work of their local domestic violence forums. The women from each have met to facilitate co-ordination, to get to know each other, to compare notes on developments in the two cities and to have enjoyable experiences together.

The Phoenix Group is an ongoing group of domestic violence survivors that has been in operation for several years and acts as a consultative body to the Westminster Domestic Violence Forum. It is sensitively facilitated by the co-ordinator of the wider forum, who is based at a local Family Service Unit. After its years of operation, the Phoenix Group is well established, respected, successful and supportive. The group started off being known as 'the Survivors' Group', but has changed its name to 'Phoenix' to give some idea of the transformations to which it has contributed, both on a personal level and as regards policy development in the area. Members say that: 'we moved from "the Survivors' Group" to "the Phoenix Group" because it is more powerful' . . . 'we are doing something practical with our experience' . . . 'as a group we have a voice – so we are heard'.

Part of the Phoenix Group's success is due to the fact that survivor involvement was built into the work of the Westminster Domestic Violence Forum from the very beginning, with funding agreed and attached, and all members of the forum were committed to it from the outset. This issue was discussed more fully in the last chapter. Thus, the aims of the main domestic violence forum always included integrating the views of abuse survivors and the commitment throughout has been that, without the incorporation of these views, the work done is likely to be incomplete and ill-informed. Members of the forum did not have to be won over to this position, as is likely to be the case in some other localities. They already subscribed to such principles and believed that, in the long-term vision of ending domestic violence, the voices of abused women themselves are key. However, the forum did not know how to put these principles into practice at the beginning and has experimented and evolved its practice in careful and sensitive ways over time.

With input from a worker from another agency who was particularly committed to working with service users, the issue was written into the budget at the beginning, as noted, even though the money involved has never been a large amount. With this money reliably put aside for survivor consultation, it was possible to establish the group with a strong commitment that the women involved should not be 'used' by the forum, but that the experience should be a constructive one for all. The forum has sometimes made use of consultants, who have knowledge and expertise in developing accountability of services to their users, in order to take advice and help from elsewhere to foster the work in Westminster. Learning from the development of the group, it is clear that, for this model to be successful, there needs to be constant, committed and honest feedback, to and fro, between the main forum and the group, and that this feedback needs to be conducted by a skilled, committed facilitator who is trusted by both sides.

The Phoenix Group has commented on, and produced reports and recommendations on, service provision in the area. To their credit, the forum and its member agencies have always responded positively and in a serious way to these recommendations and have made changes in their policy as a result. This has included work, for example, on the use of the law in domestic violence cases, on the needs of black and minority ethnic communities and on public awareness. The group and the forum have also worked on education, policing, training for agency staff, improving links between agencies and on outreach support for abused women and children. The comments and reports by the Phoenix Group have been carefully produced to provide detailed evidence and to raise questions for policy-makers on the reality of living with domestic violence. For example, the group strongly recommended that the forum do prevention work and this led directly to a joint decision by agencies in Westminster to address and develop work with male perpetrators. It also recommended that work needed to be undertaken in the education system, with the result that a comprehensive training pack has been developed for use in schools. The group participates actively in the various forum sub-groups, as discussed in the last chapter, and has made direct practical contributions to the development of domestic violence policy and practice in Westminster. It is also able to take on, in a meaningful and careful way, issues of cultural difference and the stigmatising effects of experiencing abuse, within an environment of mutual assistance.

The women in the group suggest that: 'we have support for one another and understanding as well as hearing our differences' . . . 'we're different women from different cultures and we're here to support each other'. The group has taken forward the lives of the women and their children through mutual help in ways which would have been unimaginable at the beginning.

Voice for Change

Voice for Change is an inspirational group of domestic violence survivors which has been in operation in Liverpool for more than ten years. It was established originally by two powerful survivors of violence, one of whom, a well-known and highly regarded figure in the field locally, has since sadly died. The two women originally came to the Liverpool Domestic Violence Forum to tell their stories, because they perceived rightly that their voices, and the voices of other abused women, were not being heard. The group has developed from these beginnings to become a powerful player in the domestic violence field in Liverpool. Unusually for a domestic violence survivors' forum, it has no facilitator, although it is supported and assisted by the invaluable input of the local domestic violence prevention co-ordinator.

At the beginning, the group experienced teething problems, as might be anticipated (although that stage is far in the past now), and much was expected of it by professionals, even though it did not have any workers. Over the years, Voice for Change has been situated within various different agencies and offices. There was a period when it was exploited by statutory organisations who would refer on to it many of their own domestic violence cases, in spite of the fact that the group had no money or resources. In discussions with other self-organised groups of domestic violence survivors about this issue during our study, it has become clear that this unfortunate exploiting of unfunded community groups by agencies that have a responsibility to provide services happens time and time again. Clearly, this is an outcome to be guarded against by statutory sector bodies, however desperate they may be to deal with all their own referrals, perhaps with scant or decreasing resources in their own budgets with which to do so.

Voice for Change now has its own premises and runs a variety of projects and services. It provides support for women survivors, information, consultation for agencies and campaigning. It also comments on policy and has become a service provider in its own right, running community drop-in centres. It provides a training opportunity for local counsellors, matching them to women experiencing violence who want to access counselling services. The local Crime and Disorder Audit and Strategy included consultation with Voice for Change and the group has also been involved in the evaluation of local services and campaigns, for example the Zero Tolerance public awareness campaign which was held in the city. It has provided comments and recommendations for policy development and has produced documents on what services abused women and their children need. Importantly, it has produced a Charter for Change to which various local agencies have signed up, formally committing themselves to carrying out the policy and practice reforms proposed in the Charter. Others could, perhaps, learn from this strategy of getting local organisations to agree to 'sign up' to working towards demands and suggestions put forward by survivors. Voice for Change is an outstanding example of a group of this type that has survived and prospered in the long term. This success is a tribute both to the women members and to the background support from the domestic violence prevention co-ordinator who has offered them constant inspiration and stability. The group is a testimony to what domestic violence survivors can achieve together over the long haul.

Key issues for survivors' forums

The conclusion to be reached from the experience of these various brave experiments is perhaps that, if a project to involve domestic violence survivors is set up well and facilitated sufficiently carefully, avoiding patronising responses and building towards equality with some sort of emancipatory vision to guide the endeavour, there are real possibilities for creating exciting change. In such a situation, the women involved will undoubtedly gain a great deal, building their confidence and self-respect. Policy development and change will also become possible.

In common with other participation strategies, as discussed on a general level in the previous chapter, there are many issues to be sensitively addressed if abused women are to be able to attend survivors' forums on a regular basis and if they are to be accountable in some informal way to other survivors. These issues are debated in the rest of this chapter.

One key matter to be considered is who is to serve on a domestic violence survivors' forum or advisory group. How to constitute these groups to make them at least somewhat representative is clearly an issue, notwithstanding our previous arguments about unrealistic external expectations of repre-sentativeness in user groups more generally. Being able to speak for others is particularly important for an ongoing group of this type which feeds directly into policy development. There are also important equality issues in terms of ensuring that different communities are not excluded. Formal quota representation does not seem to work well as it imposes too much of a straitjacket on the flexibility and humanity needed, but, equally, diver-sity cannot be ignored. It is all too easy for a survivors' forum to consist of white women only, for example, to the exclusion of other interests, views and experiences.

There can also be a measure of discomfort in an ongoing group, with participants sometimes coming to feel, as time goes on, that their whole life and personality have been reduced to their experience of abuse. Consultation mechanisms can make it seem as if this is all that anyone else is interested in, so that participating in them can come to feel belittling, demeaning and 'labelling'. One remedy for this may be consciously and openly to share women's positive efforts to survive, to resist and to find effective help, including for their children.

As for other consultation or participation methods, issues of safety and confidentiality need to be paramount, and this has implications for choice of venues, which need to be both accessible and safe, and for transportation to and from the survivors' forum meetings. To be a member of an established group over time can mean a certain measure of public visibility, and this can be particularly damaging, or even dangerous, for women who have escaped violent partners and who are either actually in hiding from them or who do not want their ex-abusers to know where they are.

It is important not to exploit participants in these or other ways, as discussed previously, especially where the group is expected to meet more on a long-term basis than on a short-term one. One could also ask why forum members should keep on attending over time, unless there is positive feedback and some compensation offered. Barnes *et al.* (1999) similarly emphasise that user groups require constant effort to maintain an adequate level of membership, and this problem is accentuated when the work being done becomes boring or alienating (as work with a local authority or using a bureaucratic process can often be) and when there is no recompense for the effort, energy or commitment being donated.

Payment for participants engaging in such an ongoing and committed piece of work is always the best option, although, as discussed in the last chapter, this can be payment in kind or in confidence-boosting possibilities, and may vary with local circumstances. None of the domestic violence survivors' forums discussed above have ever paid their participants in cash, although there has been reciprocity of other kinds, such as training, esteem-building and support. Few local authorities, partnership groups or inter-agency forums have resources available for payment of forum members under current circumstances. This does not mean, however, that specific resource allocation could not be built into future budgets as a matter of course, building on local and central government commitments to user accountability.

While payment is a complicated issue to resolve, reimbursement for expenses and the offering of other support to facilitate survivors taking on the tasks is a straightforward matter of agency responsibility. It is essential that resources are provided for support, training, supervision and consultancy on the one hand, and for the provision of general expenses, childcare, transport, translation/interpreting and accessibility policies on the other, to assist survivors' forum members to do the job. Working as a survivors' forum alongside an inter-agency forum is a complex role to fulfil and needs support in terms of both resources and, often, professional assistance.

An issue to be considered, for example, in an ongoing forum can be crises and personal difficulties for members over time. Groups and organisations engaged in this enterprise need to experiment and to be willing to try new approaches which may or may not work. It cannot be done quickly or half-heartedly. This is especially the case because the underlying cause that has brought participants together, namely domestic violence, is such a painful and destructive one. Partly as a result of these traumatic realities and partly because any long-term group is likely to have its ups and downs, there is sometimes, as we have noted, a tendency for groups to encounter difficulties in interactions between members. This may require support, consultancy or some other form of help with conflict resolution.

Another issue to be taken on is that, where survivors' forums have developed, they have often attempted to address issues of alienating working practices and potentially patronising or unnecessary 'committee' language usage by agencies, both of which have been raised by many other service groups (see Chapter 7). In this endeavour, they have not always, however, met with great success. One woman who had experienced violence and had been involved in many consultation exercises, including a domestic violence survivors' forum, explained to us that:

> Well, you keep trying. But, half the time, you can't understand what they are going on about. They seem to talk endlessly in circles. And half of what they say is not relevant or someone else has already said it and then they turn and smile at you and say 'what does the survivors' forum think?' What are you meant to say? But, when it does work and the survivors' forum says things they listen to, it's great.
>
> (Survivor previously active in a survivors' forum)

Domestic violence survivors' forums often have to struggle with the off-putting and uninviting nature of the task, and members may ask themselves why they bother. It can be distressing to have to battle with densely written policy documents and official jargon, replete these days with references to performance indicators and seemingly remote partnership groupings, which may appear to have little relevance to responding to immediate situations of violence. This problem can be exacerbated where there has been an elaboration by inter-agency and statutory organisations of complex strategies and protocols, often accompanied by little in the way of implementation or of real change on the ground for women experiencing violence and for their children. To deal with such issues is a hard task, and some among the small number of survivors' forums or advisory groups which exist emphasise that detailed policy analysis may be unnecessary in any case, especially if the group is principally acting as a consultative one. A better way forward, in many cases, would be for the survivors' group, instead, to develop a more overall view with examples of good and bad practice, and information on how both these would feel to women service users. However, this type of approach would clearly not be adequate if the survivors' forum was engaged in more comprehensive accountability work, checking and monitoring, for example, the practical initiatives of the wider forum.

An important element in combatting the alienating and painful impact that the policy process can have on service users is for the work of survivors' forums to contain an element of pleasure. Celebration by groups of domestic violence survivors and the enjoyment of activities together can contradict the very ethos of abuse and can be empowering in themselves for the abused women taking part. Our study found that pleasure and fun are essential if survivors' forums are to succeed, given the rather thankless task of trying to influence domestic violence policy-makers and the range of difficulties involved.

One of these difficulties which can be particularly disillusioning is how to get policy groups, forums and agencies to take the process seriously and to act upon it. Even more so than for one-off groups, ongoing women's forums sometimes feel betrayed and side-lined, when their careful contributions, perhaps made over a period of time, are ignored, even when the reason may be overwork and exhaustion on the part of policy-makers facing too many demands and scarce resources. In general, working out participation procedures which are effective and making sure they are not then overlooked can be a skilful and complex task, as discussed later in Chapter 10, and considerable commitment to the process is required from the agencies involved. In the case of survivors' forums, there needs to be a recognised way for the views of the forum to feed into the work of the main forum or agency. Importantly, in best practice, there must be an agreed protocol for then acting upon them. Interviewees in our study who had experience of domestic violence survivors' forums were usually clear that the exercise was pointless unless it led to constructive change. Co-ordinators or group representatives need to be able to advocate strongly on behalf of the survivors' group, a demanding activity which requires sensitivity, honesty and often a degree of confidence and skill at intervening in professional meetings on behalf of the group.

From the above discussions, it can be seen that there is no doubt that the facilitation or co-ordination offered to survivors' forums needs to be extremely skilled and sensitive, to take on the distressing issues involved in living with domestic violence and the difficulty of getting policy-makers to listen to women's views on an ongoing basis in a way in which they may not be used to doing. Facilitators of any sort of survivor participation process, including survivors' forums, certainly need experience and expertise in dealing with domestic violence and with the emotional complications and sensitivities involved. This is likely to include skills in supporting survivors, in responding to trauma and in dealing with complex issues of diversity and equality. Skills and abilities in running and managing groups and an understanding of group dynamics are also likely to be required, especially where an ongoing long-term survivors' forum is involved. Additionally, facilitators need an understanding of the issues involved in survivor consultation and an ability to steer issues through the policy process and to understand local authority and other structures. Ideally, such a facilitator would have good links with policy-makers in the field and be able to draw on these to enable the process. Self-advocacy survivors' forums also exist with no facilitator, although often with powerful women participants.

Thus, overall, the evidence from the study we conducted is that domestic violence survivors' forums or advisory groups can be successful, rewarding and even inspirational. But they are only able to grow in this way where they include an element of personal support and enjoyment as well as policy work, where adequate resourcing is available and, normally, where skilled facilitation is provided by an experienced facilitator who is well versed in domestic violence issues. They offer an innovatory way forward, though it is important to emphasise that they are worth engaging in only if they are able to influence services and lead to policy development – in other words, where they become more than mere consultation procedures, but, rather, devolve some influence and power to the survivors involved.

No one really knows whether survivors' forums can flourish throughout the domestic violence field, or whether they only do so in a few cases where inspiring or catalytic facilitation, support and commitment are available from the agencies involved. All involved need to learn as they go along, as these women service users point out:

> You can't run women's forums in a hurry – it takes a while, plus input and resources. It is no good trying to do it on the cheap. It needs to be a basic part of all policy and financed properly if it is to work. You have to work out how to do it and be willing to experiment.
> (Member of women's survivor group)

In some cases, we can learn from developments in other countries. The Toronto Woman Abuse Council in Toronto, Canada, for example, is a long-standing, senior level inter-agency collaboration, which plays a key role in service and policy development in Toronto. It has dealt with the issue of survivor input and participation very successfully and has, for many years, operated an Accountability Committee. This Committee consists of abuse survivors, and provides input and feedback on all initiatives undertaken. There is no problem, apparently, in attaining a consistent and committed response from survivors on the committee, perhaps indicating the respect in which the Woman Abuse Council is held. Participants are expected to be at a stage in their own recovery from trauma where they are able to take on the work, although the organisation recognises that this is a complex issue (as discussed earlier) and may vary from woman to woman. Members receive childcare expenses and a small honorarium. The Accountability Committee has also led a project to produce a moving document on 'Sharing our Stories' (Woman Abuse Council of Toronto, 1999). The

Council is committed to being accountable to this Committee, which makes deciding comments on all work undertaken and has the final word on policies to be adopted (Hague *et al.*, 2001a). In these ways, it surpasses anything we have in this country and provides an interesting model to work towards. There are other international examples of abused women's groups to which policy-makers are directly (but usually informally) accountable. The Duluth Domestic Abuse Intervention Project in Minnesota, for example, has developed a complex, co-ordinated community response to domestic violence, including perpetrators' programmes, the tracking of cases through the criminal justice system and community development, all responsible to groups of survivors (Pence and Shepard, 1999). In these examples, services have moved on from basic consultation to being directly accountable to women survivors.

In summary, in this chapter, we have discussed the innovatory work of domestic violence forums and advisory groups in the UK and beyond, and the positives, sensitivities and difficulties involved. They offer a helpful way forward and are growing in popularity, particularly in regard to advising inter-agency domestic violence forums and policy groups. While they can be used as a solely consultative exercise, they also have the potential to give service users real power in the policy process and to lead towards accountability of services to survivors, as in the international examples described above.

Chapter 9

Further innovatory practice

Women's Aid and women's advocacy organisations and campaigns

In this chapter, we move on from considering domestic violence survivors' forums to discuss survivor representation through Women's Aid and refuge groups and through the local, national and international campaigning, advocacy and lobbying of women's organisations. In the UK, Women's Aid and other women's advocacy and support groups work closely with women who have experienced domestic violence and with their children, and have always had policies of raising their voices, as discussed throughout this book. In terms of both basic consultation and broader participation strategies, there are ways in which the work of women's organisations and self-activity is particularly pertinent, especially in terms of sharing power between women who are survivors and those who are not.

Women's Aid and other women's projects employ many domestic violence survivors and ex-service users as volunteers, workers and managers (as explored in Part 2 and further discussed in Chapter 10). Where ex-service users participate in agencies directly as employees or within management structures, they are likely to have at least some power in the operation of that agency and may also be able to take a policy-making role. In some senses, then, this can be the most developed type of survivor involvement. Within refuges and outreach projects, women using the service may also take a role in the day-to-day running of the project and in publicity, training and education work, as discussed in Chapter 5, and may be able to impact on, or exert some control over, this work.

In terms of influencing wider domestic violence policy-making and the role of statutory and voluntary agencies, Women's Aid and other women's projects play a key advocacy role representing abused women's views. They also conduct campaigning work in which abused women themselves play a crucial role. Further, on a local level, women's organisations are engaged in other ways of getting women's voices heard, for example, within inter-agency forums and partnership groupings. In this area of work, consultation with service users (through refuge organisations) remains the most common method, as for other forms of user involvement, even though, as we have emphasised throughout this book, it is also the most limited.

Structured involvement of Women's Aid and refuge groups as a 'conduit' for survivors' views

Looking at consultation methods first then, it might seem obvious that effective ways of involving abused women can usefully take place using the conduit of refuge organisations and specialist women's domestic violence services. In fact, it can appear to be so obvious that, as noted previously, many domestic violence forums refer to the mere presence of women's refuges in their ranks to suggest that consultation with service users is taking place, even where no such consultation has been suggested, discussed, agreed or carried out. Just by being there, women's refuge and outreach organisations give forums credibility, and inappropriate claims about survivor involvement may then be bandied about (often in good faith) by members. In our recent study, we came across repeated examples of this happening.

Nevertheless, where consultation is actually agreed and carried out through this route (rather than constituting wishful thinking by the forum or agency concerned), this can be an effective and efficient way of doing it. The advantage is that women using projects can be directly and easily consulted within a familiar environment by skilled refuge and outreach workers, who are expert in domestic violence work. Workers are then able to provide support when women being consulted want or need it, as part of the process. They are also in a good position to feed the results back to the forum, which they are probably already attending anyway. A disadvantage is that workers may (often inadvertently) influence their residents' views so that results are skewed. It is also the case that such consultation is unlikely to uncover problems about the refuge provision itself. Additionally, the only women involved are those who are already in contact with Women's Aid or other refuge and outreach projects. This could mean that women suffering abuse, but not using Women's Aid, are excluded from the process and that their voices remain silenced.

Further, many refuge organisations are already stretched to their limits in terms of running their services, so that passing on women service users' views to inter-agency forums and to policy-makers may not be a priority – or may fall off the agenda altogether due to overwork. Indeed, few refuge workers have the spare time or energy available to enable them to view this work enthusiastically as an important part of their brief, or to encourage them to engage in it all. One study found, for example, that, of seventy women survivors interviewed in various areas of the country, only two had any knowledge whatsoever of multi-agency domestic violence work in their own locality. In particular, almost all of those who were living in Women's Aid refuges knew absolutely nothing of their local domestic violence inter-agency forum, even where the refuge organisation itself was active within it (Hague *et al.*, 1996). The refuge workers had either not thought of involving their residents or had no time to do so.

However, consultation with women in refuges on specific subjects is now becoming more common (especially through research interviews or surveys of refuge residents, as will be further discussed later). As regards wider liaison with inter-agency forums, a few women's refuge and outreach organisations have tried to conduct systematic, organised consultation, often by convening special one-off groups of abused women. Such groups may consist of residents, ex-residents, or users of outreach services or helplines, who are then able to comment on policy and service provision, sometimes as a logical extension of the work which refuge organisations already do in representing abused women's and children's views. These groups may discuss very specific local policy and service developments, and may also both comment on the work of the local inter-agency forum itself and feed ideas into it. While specially convened groups of this nature, established through refuge and outreach services, can take a key role in advising domestic violence forums and agencies, they can be hard to organise in that women residents are likely to be in severe personal crisis and may have little time to engage in such activities, in addition to everything else. However, ex-residents may be able to contribute more easily. Abused women using refuge and outreach services can also advise on the work of forums and agencies through already existing mechanisms, rather than specially established ones. For example, most women in refuges are expected to attend refuge house meetings which could discuss wider policy issues on occasion and then send the resultant ideas to forum meetings.

Overall, then, Women's Aid and other women's support, outreach and refuge organisations are often in a position to represent abused women's voices in a structured way to other agencies (even if they do so less often at present than they could), and to act as a channel, backwards and forwards, for information exchange. Domestic violence forums or agencies are thus able to ask groups of survivors directly for their opinions on specific subjects, through the medium of the refuge or women's group. The views expressed can then be fed back to the forum or agency by Women's Aid representatives so that the 'conduit' process is complete in both directions.

This way of reaching abused women is used in various localities by domestic violence services, particularly by multi-agency forums, in order to access abused women's views. However, Women's Aid and refuge workers should not be expected to do this work routinely, with no arrangements in place to assist them to do so, and no acknowledgement and recompense for the extra time, effort and energy required. Further, consultation of this type may lead to criticisms of funders being voiced by the women consulted, which refuges may not wish to have attributed to themselves if their financial position is precarious. Thus, this approach needs to be carefully used. It also needs both to be formally agreed and facilitated by the agencies or forums involved and to be properly structured in order to be successful. Refuge organisations are usually overworked and rarely have spare time or resources to conduct this work, as noted above. Thus, it needs to be an agreed and structured principle of operation for the relevant inter-agency forum or project, and for the refuge or women's group involved.

This is likely to have resource implications. Women's organisations clearly need to be compensated in some way if they conduct consultation and advisory work on behalf of other agencies. With the current emphasis on user involvement in legislation and policy development, Women's Aid and refuge-based support services that represent abused women's views may be asked to engage in one consultative exercise after another. These days, they may similarly be asked to contribute to one research project after another, seeking the opinions of refuge workers and abuse survivors, so that, even with the best will in the world, 'questionnaire fatigue' can set in. With the ongoing lack of secure and comprehensive funding for 24-hour emergency refuge services (despite the contribution of the Supporting People programme from 2003) and the general resource shortage in this field, it is not possible for these services continually to conduct such work without payment or recognition.

Campaigning, community arts and general liaison with agencies representing abused women

Structured and agreed consultation through refuge organisations is just one aspect of the more general consultative, lobbying and advising role carried out by the Women's Aid federations, and by women's groups and other agencies that represent domestic violence survivors, including black women's advocacy and advice organisations, for example the Asian Women's Resource Centre in the London Borough of Brent. Women's Aid, in particular, and other refuge projects represent and advocate on behalf of abused women and their children locally and nationally, and have done so with increasing frequency and influence over recent years (see Women's Aid, 2001/2). In fact, liaison with agencies that represent women and children experiencing domestic violence has been identified by the Home Office and by research studies on multi-agency domestic violence work as vital to effective inter-agency practice and policy development (see Hague et al., 1996; Harwin et al., 1999; Home Office, 1999; James-Hanman, 2000). Importantly, this work includes liaison with women service users. Women's services and the activist women's movement in general now occupy a key role in facilitating policy and service development across the board.

Throughout the country, Women's Aid and other national organisations collect, collate, produce and publicise information about domestic violence and abused women's views on both a local level and also in the national and international arena. The Women's Aid federations across the UK are able to commission or conduct research surveys of users accessing their networks of services nationally, and they produce many publications, reports and briefing papers. Thus, while women's refuge, support and advocacy organisations represent abused women's views locally, the federations and other nationally based women's organisations represent these voices and needs on both a local and a wider level, through national networks, conferences and sub-groups, and through policy and advisory work with local and central government. A variety of other organisations are also able to represent abused women's views nationally and internationally and to advocate on their behalf. Imkaan, for instance, works with the national network of Asian women's refuges, producing briefing papers and conducting research on issues of relevance.

A powerful way to raise voices otherwise unheard is through direct campaigning, and many distinctive women's campaigning organisations exist. An example, as we have noted previously, is provided by Southall Black Sisters, which represents abused women in both the local and the national arena and conducts campaigning and awareness-raising work on behalf, particularly, of women and children from minority ethnic communities facing abuse. The campaigning messages of Southall Black Sisters also contribute to international initiatives and their pioneering work is known in a variety of other countries (see, for example, in relation to the new South Africa, Park *et al.*, 2000). Thus, campaigns are an important way to access the voices of abused women, particularly, in this case, those demanding justice and improvements in services and policy. Some of the best and most successful campaigns on domestic violence have been mounted over the years to fight for justice for individual domestic violence survivors, for example Balwant Kaur, Kiranjit Ahluwalia, Sara Thornton and Emma Humphreys, all of whom have taken an active part in the campaigns where possible. A variety of campaigns against rape have been conducted over the years, all with many members who are rape survivors themselves.

Campaigns may use traditional methods of demonstrations, petitions, letter-writing and so on. However, relevant organisations may extend beyond activist women's projects and make use, more widely, of community action involving members of the public and local women who have experienced violence. Community theatre, art and poetry workshops can provide a creative and imaginative way to reach abused women as part of awareness-raising and training for professionals, or as a technique for campaigning and for influencing policy-makers. Drama can work particularly powerfully in this context. For example, 'Legislative Theatre' groups, connected to the 'Theatre of the Oppressed' movement of Agusto Boal, sometimes engage in innovative dramatic collaborations, where skilled actors work with community groups to construct pieces of drama which are then used to influence policy-makers and to feed directly into policy-making (as practised, for example, by Them Wifeys with women in Newcastle). In another example, we were told in our study of community-based projects in which young domestic violence survivors in a locality were developing presentations through local theatre groups that powerfully challenged community norms.

Overall, there are many creative routes for the voices of survivors to feed into activist or campaigning approaches (when these are defined in the broadest sense). The movement against violence against women is a wide-ranging and complex one (see, e.g. Dobash and Dobash, 1992), operating on many different levels. In general, it is characterised by active campaigning by women for women and, as discussed previously, has always attempted to involve grass-roots organisations and survivors. It has well-developed theories and understandings of the empowerment of women experiencing violence and of the collective strength of abused women and children.

Campaigning and lobbying work of this nature extends not only nationally, but also internationally. After so many years of inaction on violence against women, the voices of survivors now inform initiatives across the globe. These voices are frequently raised – and heard – at international gatherings on violence against women and, via grass-roots activity, feed into global work through the United Nations and other bodies (see, e.g. Davies, 1994; UNICEF, 1997). For example, the 1998 classification by the United Nations of rape in war as a war crime followed intensive grass-roots activity by women's groups and by women who had experienced abuse throughout the world, but particularly in developing countries and in areas experiencing conflict.

Thus, in this chapter, we have discussed ways of using Women's Aid and other women's organisations to act as a conduit for abused women's views. This is a way of conducting consultation and advisory work which can be particularly beneficial and we have considered the advantages and disadvantages of the approach. Certainly, our study found that it can be very effective as a way of getting women's voices heard although it still fits into the 'consultation' end of the spectrum of survivor participation, rather than moving towards user power and control. We have also discussed wider ways to involve survivors including women's advocacy and campaigning organisations, women's direct campaigns and activity in the activist movement, and abused women taking a role as employees or managers in women's services, specifically. (The latter issue is discussed in a more general way in the next chapter.)

Chapter 10

Other methods of survivor participation and getting agencies to take action

In the last two chapters, we have discussed some of the new methods being tried out to achieve survivor representation. These include domestic violence forums or advisory groups, structured representation through women's projects and the role of national and local campaigning and lobbying organisations in representing abused women's views. However, there is a wide variety of other methods which are currently in use. We discuss these in this chapter and also consider how to convert the results of participation processes into action and policy change.

Women's focus groups

We hear a great deal about focus groups these days, even though the term is rarely defined properly or used in its original sense (Greenbaum, 2000; Krueger, 2000). For the present Government, their use has become something of a mantra. Focus groups are a popular policy option in attempting to gather diverse views to inform policy-making of all types. Thus, it is almost inevitable that they should also be used in domestic violence work.

In the past few years, focus groups of domestic violence service users have been convened in a few local areas to represent women's views within the policy process. Such groups can be used to consider various aspects of policy or inter-agency work, to comment on specific policy developments and to advise on survivors' groups in general and on how to improve consultative mechanisms. They can also comment on wider developments in the domestic violence field. However, they are firmly positioned within the 'consultation' end of the range of user involvement strategies and rarely move beyond this.

A recent example of focus groups being used in this field is provided by the London Borough of Newham, which has conducted a domestic violence consultative process of this type. A few other localities have carried out general focus group consultation on behalf of inter-agency forums and, in others, specialised focus groups with, for example, black and minority ethnic women have also been held to identify specific relevant issues, gaps in service, attitudes to refuges and other services and areas for policy improvement.

Focus groups on domestic violence issues can be hard to organise, partly because of the security and safety issues involved. Transport to and from the meetings and the use of accessible and safe venues are vital, so that the women participating are not placed in any danger from past or present violent partners. Groups need to be conducted regularly, for example for a day or half-day once every six months, and there needs to be attention to diversity of membership. Focus groups in the true sense consist of women who do not know each other, so that careful and expert group leadership is likely to be required due to the sensitivity of the issues being addressed.

The evidence from our research and from localities where such groups have been attempted is that they need to be conducted by skilled facilitators, who have been carefully briefed and who are aware of – and experienced in dealing with – domestic violence issues (as discussed in the chapter on survivors' forums (Chapter 8)). From our study, it was clear that such groups work best where they are tied in with local authority equalities units, domestic violence forums or women's projects in the voluntary sector in some way, rather than with private companies commissioned to undertake market research. Certainly, if other external agencies are involved, it is preferable for focus groups of this type to be conducted by commissioned researchers from the public arena who specialise in abuse issues, rather than being run by commercial, profit-making concerns, partly because safety and confidentiality must remain to the fore.

Additionally to the use of transport and of safe and accessible venues, payment for the women attending is a priority in this case, as for other types of focus groups. Similarly, the provision of childcare, expenses and interpreting or translating facilities where required is essential (in the same way as for survivors' advisory forums). As for other types of consultation, too, the experience of participating needs to be rewarding and enjoyable, and there also need to be processes in place whereby support can be provided if traumatic memories are evoked for the women. All the various methods that are in use for raising abused women's voices need a mechanism for feeding into the policy-making process, and this is equally the case for translating focus group results into action and policy. Agencies may already have such mechanisms in place in regard to other professionally-run groups (for example, for wider consultation by Crime and Disorder and other partnerships, all of which require community involvement and are then expected to feed the results back into policy).

Special mechanisms

In this section, we consider some of the various individually tailored possibilities that exist for involving abused women in policy and service development, rather than the more general methods discussed previously. In some local areas, specific mechanisms for hearing service users' views have been tried out with considerable success. For example, the chairperson or other officers of the local domestic violence forum in some localities have held consultation meetings with women's support groups or refuge residents. In such situations, women are able to feed in their views directly within a fairly sympathetic environment, and officers who have conducted such consultations are often deeply moved by the testimonies and experiences related. Being brought face to face with 'reality' in this way has, in various cases, led to the professional taking up the issues concerned with renewed and informed commitment and zeal.

Similarly, regular or one-off public meetings of abused women with senior local managers and policy-makers may be held, where the latter are held to account for the quality and delivery of services, and may also seek participants' views on possible improvements. Our study found that, where such meetings have been held, they have apparently been powerful occasions in which senior or chief executives have been asked in a constructive way by service users to account for, and justify, detailed aspects of service delivery.

Specialised consultation can also be carried out with particular groups of survivors, such as women from specific minority ethnic communities, as a structured and agreed project of the forum or agency. The domestic violence forum may need, for example, to be informed about the needs of Chinese or Turkish women in a locality, or there may be a specific new piece of policy on which it is vital to obtain women's views and which will affect certain minority groups differentially. In best practice, such meetings should be carefully and constructively conducted in a forward-looking manner, rather than as a necessary formality. Several London forums have sought views on domestic violence from different groups, for instance of black, refugee or asylum-seeking women. One way to do this is to hold meetings between the inter-agency forum or individual agency and local women's advocacy organisations, who may then set up a special meeting, often on their premises, with women abuse survivors. This type of exercise clearly must be carried out in culturally sensitive ways, with interpretation and translation available, and meetings needto be held in venues that are sympathetic to the issue. Facilitators ideally need to be of a similar ethnic or community background to participants, and preferably able to speak the appropriate community languages.

Great care needs to be taken in organising such meetings as regards issues of confidentiality, safety and the dominant view of domestic violence among the community in question. It is often good practice to carry out consultation with a specific community group but, in the case of intimate family matters and domestic violence, it has to be recognised that to raise these matters, and to name the existence of violence, may cut across the views and wishes of some community leaders (see Southall Black Sisters, 1990). One acceptable way round this problem, which has been utilised by a number of projects, can be if domestic violence issues are brought up in the context of other services (e.g. a drop-in morning with crèche provision or a general meeting on women's safety). These complex issues need careful handling by women from the communities concerned who speak the locally used languages and who perhaps can draw personal support from other specialist women's groups also familiar with the relevant community and cultural issues. In part, these complexities are due to the ongoing marginalisation of many minority ethnic communities and to potential racism in service delivery and in UK society as a whole. These painful realities further complicate cultural issues that are already very complicated, especially for translocated cultural groups (see James-Hanman, 1995; Mama, 1996).

For disabled women who are abuse survivors, issues of full accessibility and safety will be paramount in any form of user involvement. It is all too easy for non-disabled policy-makers and practitioners to overlook issues of disability in the participative strategies they adopt, although things are perhaps improving in this respect currently. Again, focused consultation with specific groups or organisations, including those for deaf women, can be useful, but it is important to remember that disabled women also need a voice in all user participation, of whatever type, as an automatic part of good practice. Disabled respondents in our study warned against specialised consultation with disabled women that results in their being 'ghettoised' into a specialised area, and often then subjected to marginalisation. Issues of confidentiality, sensitivity and accessibility (in its broadest sense) exist across the board, for instance for lesbian groups. In all these instances, the safety and protection of the specialised group of women who are participating must be paramount.

Surveys, questionnaires and research projects

Agencies and inter-agency forums sometimes make use of exit question-naires for service users who have finished using the service. These can play a key part in project evaluation, now requested for most funded organisa-tions. Similarly, organisations may seek user views through the routine monitoring of service use required by funders and managements, but possibly expanded and developed more fully. Consultation is also possible through the medium of user surveys, satisfaction questionnaires and so on, as is standard practice for other types of services and consultative struc-tures. In this way, services can at best be effectively (rather than cosmetically) evaluated, by those who have used them and who thus have the opportunity to give their views privately and confidentially.

However, the results of service user evaluations of this type still need to be fed into the planning and development process within the organisation in question so as to lead to improved practice. Thus, as for all types of participation, a method needs to exist to translate the results of surveys and questionnaires into action. Very often, though, an implementation strategy is lacking, so that surveys and other research with service users and ex-users may lead to the production of a report, but frequently go no further, thus negating the effort of all those involved. This issue is currently receiving considerable attention, for example by specialist umbrella groups dedicated to research dissemination, such as Making Research Count, Research in Practice and SCIE (the Social Care Institute for Excellence). The latter has user knowledge as an equal part of the input it values, along-side formal research findings and audit information. Domestic violence is on the agenda for all these organisations.

Specialised research projects to seek specific women's views have been conducted in some London boroughs looking at the needs of black or disabled women (James-Hanman, 1994; Greenwich Asian Women's Project, 1995; Brent Asian Women's Resource Centre, 2000/1), and this type of survey approach can enhance consultation with such groups, as discussed above. Broader research studies of abused women's views and wishes may also be conducted, across a locality or nationally, by local authorities, health trusts, Crime and Disorder or other partnerships, or Women's Aid. Such studies may also be commissioned from university and other research groups. One example is the previously cited *Routes to Safety* research recently conducted for Women's Aid nationally by the Centre for the Study of Safety and Well-being at the University of Warwick (Humphreys and Thiara, 2002). Specialist 'violence against women' research groups and researchers now exist in a variety of higher education establishments. These research centres or individual researchers have developed expertise in domestic violence issues and in interviewing survivors of abuse. The use of researchers with this expertise to conduct research with domestic violence service users is helpful, due to the sensitivity of the task and the need for mature researchers able to deal with issues of violence.

Internet consultation

A new way of seeking the views of domestic violence survivors which we will undoubtedly hear more about in the future is via the Internet. Electronic discussion with women who have experienced domestic violence is a new and developing area (in the United States, for example). It offers advantages of privacy and confidentiality, to a large extent. Names and postal addresses do not have to be revealed and consultation can take place over a wide geographical area, although safety issues exist for women living with their abusers or for those who are using computers (either public or private) which are not secure. Access to the website concerned also needs the highest level of security, but this is usually in place.

Women's Aid, the Hansard Society and the All Party Parliamentary Group on Domestic Violence held the first consultation by means of the Internet with women experiencing domestic abuse in the UK in 2000 (see Bossey and Coleman, 2000). This exercise is discussed further in a contribution by Nicola Harwin, the Director of the Women's Aid Federation of England, included in the Epilogue to this book. This is now being followed up by other consultations, including one with children who have experienced domestic violence, in 2003. The latter consultation is also being organised by the All Party Parliamentary Group on Domestic Violence in conjunction with the major children's charities and is funded by the BBC. Additionally, at least one Internet site (moderated by survivors) now exists for those who have been abused. This site is both a supportive chat room and a forum that can be used for discussion of policy issues.

Feeding into effective policy development: regular feedback, service standards and protocols

Most of the methods for involving abused women that have been discussed in this chapter have concentrated principally on consultation, rather than more thoroughgoing participation. Consulting with and getting information from service uses can be achieved by one of the methods discussed above. However, for domestic violence survivors to have any power in the policy process, their views need to lead to action, as we have constantly reaffirmed. And effectively feeding women's perspectives and the results of participation exercises into the policy process can be problematic.

Survivors interviewed for our study were critical of participation processes which led nowhere at all. One woman had this to say:

> It's not good unless consultation with women translates into actual policy and change. . . . So often views are sought and then – what do the agencies do with the views you've sought out? Ignore them. With real participation/accountability – things actually change as a result. The power of survivors needs to be real, real power. And it's tough to do for everyone. We don't have the answer yet.
>
> (Woman survivor)

One standard method of attempting to make sure women's voices are heard and acted on is through the incorporation of a regular feedback and consultation slot at decision-making meetings, which can then become a standard feature of all policy development. Thus, feedback from, and responses to, service users can be made an agreed part of agendas at official meetings of agencies at management and policy-making level, and at inter-agency forums. With an agreed procedure for reporting information from domestic violence survivors, the basics have been provided for agencies then to act on this information. However, clear issues have to be addressed about how such feedback is conducted and by whom.

In some localities, survivors may be able to influence their local forum and agencies directly by attending or by sending representatives. But, as discussed in Chapter 7, it may not be appropriate for individual service users to attend agency meetings, although this will vary with circumstances. Feedback can be conducted by development workers, forum co-ordinators or other specialist officers instead. In one example, members of an inter-agency forum that contributed to our research had developed an effective system in which workers reported back to the forum on survivors' behalf, as follows:

> Frontline staff represent the views of abused women in a principled way. In our experience, many abused women do not wish to be labelled as such and wish issues to be carried forward on their behalf whilst they pursue their own lives. The forum seeks to ensure that all community groups and agencies which represent survivors are invited to meetings and feed in and are kept fully informed as well.
>
> (Inter-agency forum member)

Workers or group facilitators may be able to report back in this way extremely effectively and, in so doing, bring reality and clarity to the resulting work. However, this method can be patronising in that service users are 'spoken on behalf of' rather than speaking for themselves. Where issues of ethnicity, sexuality and disability are concerned, this can be a particularly inappropriate outcome. And, sometimes, the outcome in any case seems to play into the 'meeting ethos' of agencies rather than to contribute to action and change.

While service user views can be introduced into policy development by one of the methods discussed above, or by a combination of several, the next stage of using the information (that has been successfully fed in) to achieve change can be even harder to achieve. One way to raise the profile of survivors' voices can be to establish agreed procedures that policy-makers are required to abide by (as we discussed in Chapter 7), so that input from women users is expected, is given authority, substance and official 'space' – and is then routinely acted upon. Forums and agencies may develop specific protocols that embed such processes into their procedure and working practice, for example. Protocols of this type need to provide not just for feedback at meetings, but for effective use of that feedback in policy-making, with agreements in place to govern this and to make sure that it happens. The agencies in the Liverpool Domestic Violence Forum, for example, have 'signed up' to agree to abide by recommendations from the survivors' group, as we discussed previously. Other inter-agency forums have agreed protocols to govern their activities, including overall standards and details of the involvement of survivors. Individual agencies may have such standards written into their service level agreements or other working policies.

In our study, we found a variety of examples of policy-makers and managers acting on information from survivors in a committed way, even where protocols to do so had not been developed. Members of one forum described listening to women and children and responding to their identified needs as a most empowering process in which they saw their own commitment as key. They described their work as follows:

> For example, survivors said that the forum must work with perpetrators if domestic violence is to be prevented in the long term. So we took on to do this in a principled way. Or survivors said all women experiencing domestic violence need to be told how well they're doing to build up their self-esteem and confidence. This is now incorporated into the DVF emotional support guidelines. Black and minority ethnic women have told us that domestic violence sounds like physical violence on its own in some other languages so now we are addressing that . . . it's all a dynamic, backwards and forwards process.
>
> (Agency manager and forum co-ordinator)

Another forum development worker discussed setting up a Users' Action Group, which had strongly influenced the forum to emphasise the urgency of appropriate responses from all the agencies involved and to provide appropriate training. This had enabled them to produce a crisis support pack for frontline practitioners, together with publicity information listing emergency contact numbers, safety preparation and legal advice. In yet another forum, the members stressed that user accountability is:

> a crucial part of our strategy. User involvement and being accountable is vital to our work, otherwise the forum's strategy becomes a meaningless exercise.

This forum was in the process of developing consultative groups of abused women on a county-wide basis. These groups were participating in the implementation of awareness-raising and service development and were also developing consultative work with children. In a further locality, abused women met regularly with a Community Initiatives Worker, and all policy development was done with women's input. For example, when the local forum had wanted to produce publicity, women experiencing violence were asked what they thought should be emphasised and, when the social services department was drawing up good practice guidelines, they directly involved the women service users. In both cases, the outcomes were then acted upon.

Where such mechanisms have become an automatic part of good practice, some workers pointed out to us that there can be sensitivities to take on board in terms of an overenthusiasm for the task. For example, co-ordinators of two domestic violence forums to whom we spoke explained that the first issue is to find out whether survivors want to be involved in the first place and, if so, at what stage. They compared this process to buying a washing machine, where what you want is good, reliable service, not to have to go out and be consulted about it. Most people probably expect to receive a good service of this type in other areas of life also – and then be done with it. Again, then, it is vital that abused women are not pressured or forced to be involved unless they want to be. Agencies and forums need to be aware of the dangers of pushing service users into feeling that they must be available for consultation duties, for example, even when they are trying to do so sensitively. The power of agency workers as gatekeepers can never be overestimated. For service users, feeling pressed into consultative roles is a likely outcome if service provision and delivery appear to be in any way dependent on this happening. Even subtle pressure can result in abused women feeling forced to help out in order to receive services.

However, while the forum workers quoted above were adamant about these issues, they also considered that:

> On the other hand, we do believe *all* services *must* be founded on service user involvement but remembering that what we believe isn't always what service users believe. In order to be accountable to abused women, we need to set standards for all agencies, with penalties for non-compliance.

Agreed protocols for converting consultation and participation methods into policy, and the development of service standards as a result, are key. Protocols and standards that all member agencies abide by, and joint understandings of the importance of survivor involvement and consultation, carried out in a principled way, are important ways forward for the future. Multi-agency forums and agencies can usefully embed these principles into their policies and operation – and also into their hearts and minds.

Doing the work: abused women as workers, managers and volunteers

There are many other ways in which domestic violence service users or ex-users and other abuse survivors can participate in the provision of

services and take an active part in their development, management, operation and delivery. A few of these possibilities are explored here.
Importantly, women's self-organisation is a vital way forward in which
abused women control their own projects, where appropriate. Self-help
groups and advocacy projects consisting solely of abuse survivors exist in
various localities, but few have a powerful role in local policy-making.
Similarly, it is vital that women survivors are in a position actually to
propose and design services and also to participate in, or control, the design
of consultative and other strategies to involve service users, rather than
have these imposed from above. It is significant that most of the mechanisms which are currently being tried and which we have discussed in this
book were designed by professionals, sometimes with some input from
service users and other survivors, but usually not. Survivors have been the
'object' of the exercise, not its 'subject' or guiding hand. This is a telling
lack.

One of the most important ways in which domestic violence service
ex-users and other abused women can be significantly involved in the work
of agencies and policy-makers is as managers or workers. Many domestic
violence survivors work for organisations which deal with domestic violence and they may feel able to speak out about their experiences, as we
have suggested throughout this book. It was repeatedly pointed out to us
in our study that survivors are represented in almost all relevant agencies,
multi-agency forums and committees.

As far as users and ex-users of services are concerned, many are also
involved in the management of projects, sit on management committees
and take on management roles, as we have noted previously, where their
understandings of the issues at hand can add depth to the process and may
complement the skills of other members. While these methods are used
most extensively in the voluntary sector, statutory organisations are also
beginning to be receptive to mechanisms to involve user or ex-user representatives in management structures. This issue is somewhat contentious,
however, as was discussed in some detail in Chapter 5, but offers a way
forward for involving survivors in policy formulation. Women service users
and ex-users may also be in a position to contribute to the day-to-day
running of projects and agencies. While this is clearly the case for women's
refuge and outreach services, where abused women often take an active
role in the running of the project as volunteers, it can also be the case for
other agencies, where their expertise and knowledge about domestic
violence can be a useful resource on which the agency can draw on an
everyday basis. The employment of domestic violence survivors or ex-
service users as workers or volunteers means that they can sometimes
contribute directly to the wider policy process.

In some projects, survivors of abuse may take on a more formal role as
trained volunteers. The Croydon One Stop Partnership, for example, was

fronted in the past by women 'friends' who were survivors of abuse, and this system will be continued in a revamping and relaunching of the project that are underway at the time of writing. The organisation brings together all the relevant agencies so that women and children experiencing abuse do not have to travel from one office to another in the quest for help. The expanded project will include three new specialist support workers and will be sited in larger and improved premises. It will encompass a successful advocacy project for domestic violence survivors, presently funded by the Home Office Crime Reduction Programme on Violence Against Women. An education support group for women will also be launched.

During our study, the friends welcomed women approaching the agency for help and conducted initial interviews with them, sometimes over cups of tea. Women we spoke with who had used this service said that they had found it deeply supportive to arrive, possibly nervously, at the project, only to be welcomed by someone with whom they could immediately identify. The friends then referred each woman on to the appropriate service (the police, housing, a solicitor and so on), all of which were under the same roof in a safe venue. This set-up will continue in the new, larger project.

The friends are crucial to the success of the project, which has attracted some acclaim. Attention has been specifically focused on the provision of support and considerable amounts of training for them, and on team and group building, which has enabled the workers to develop their professional skills and extend their expertise. Childcare, support and expenses are available. In the words of two of the friends, whom we interviewed, they form the 'glue' or the 'building blocks' of the project, holding it together. The friends both strongly supported the project at the time of the study and were proud of the work that they were conducting.

Women who have experienced domestic violence can also feed into specific or single pieces of work that an agency or forum is doing, as indicated previously, rather than having to be involved all the time. For example, there may be a one-off project on the go, which survivors can become part of for a specified period of time. Abused women often contribute to the production of leaflets, booklets, posters and other publicity materials (as already noted in specific relation to Women's Aid projects). They may sometimes, for instance, comment on samples of possible designs, suggest or advise on content and decide between different possibilities. In some cases, abused women and children have designed materials themselves completely, or have controlled the content produced by professional designers. In the Wearside Women in Need project, for example, women survivors of violence have written, designed and overseen the production of publicity materials. A particularly active forum also told us about a public awareness campaign they had run, during which survivors had played an active role in media interviews with the local and national press, radio and television. They explained that, in doing this, they had recognised the importance of protecting the women involved and said that they had:

> succeeded in retaining an unusual amount of editorial control to ensure that the women were comfortable with the articles and programmes involved.

Similarly, women experiencing violence have frequently contributed to or designed domestic violence awareness training for professionals in conjunction with trainers. They may also deliver it directly. Where abused women do this kind of work, it is of course of some importance that they are themselves trained and compensated, and are not exploited as unpaid labour. Women survivors of domestic violence are often also able to contribute to conferences and seminars, to give speeches and testimonies about their experiences, to participate in theatre pieces and to give talks to agencies.

Women who have experienced violence or used relevant services and who have taken on these types of duties may go on to engage in professional training and career development as a result, as discussed previously. Some in the field regard this as unwelcome professionalisation, as we have noted, in that survivors often then enter the very world they may previously have criticised as service users. However, the empowering possibilities for the individuals concerned and the authenticity of the resultant practice responses are clearly enhanced.

Which methods work for which agencies?

Most of the participation and consultation methods that have been discussed can be used both by inter-agency forums and by individual statutory agencies and partnerships, although some are more suitable for one arena than others. For example, ongoing domestic violence survivors' forums or advisory groups are most used by inter-agency forums and partnership groupings. Mechanisms for seeking user views on specific services offered (for example, exit questionnaires and user satisfaction surveys) are self-evidently most used by service provider agencies. General liaison by the statutory sector with agencies representing abused women (e.g. women's support groups, campaigns and refuge organisations) is to be recommended across the board.

In terms of specific policy development, the active involvement of Women's Aid and other women's services to represent abused women's voices and to act as a conduit for information exchange is important for all levels of involvement, and needs to be agreed, and if possible resourced, as discussed previously. Women's focus groups and other specialised groups (e.g. of older or disabled women) are also increasingly used within consultation processes by statutory organisations, and the future may bring a much-increased use of Internet methods.

For refuge and women's support and outreach services, the issues are rather different. They are more often the agencies being consulted than the agencies doing the consultation, and their involvement in raising survivors' voices is of key importance to policy-makers in general. In almost all refuge groups, on an overall level, it is true to say that women who have experienced domestic violence are represented as professionals among volunteers, staff or management and can sometimes speak on behalf of other survivors.

As we have discussed throughout, refuge groups have always attempted to involve women residents and ex-residents in the running and management of their projects. There is some evidence that this has decreased slightly in recent years, with greater professionalisation and administrative demands, and it may be helpful for refuge projects to consider developing new methods to achieve the full involvement of service users, as we discussed in Chapter 5. In general, however, refuge organisations and women's advocacy and support groups continue to offer a creative and radical approach to this painful subject, supported by the loose-knit global movement (Dobash and Dobash, 1992; United Nations, 1995), which, to different degrees in every nation and region of the world, challenges men's violence to women and works towards a world where such violence will have disappeared into the past.

Professionals who have experienced domestic violence

Finally, an issue which emerged over and again in the study and to which we have constantly returned throughout this book, is the indisputable fact that considerable numbers of practitioners, managers, policy-makers and activists working on abuse issues have personal experience of domestic violence, either as adults or as child witnesses of such violence in their original families. This is a painful and emotive issue that has rarely attracted attention or acknowledgement until now.

This book therefore seeks to highlight the contribution that has been made throughout the development of domestic violence provision over the last thirty years by relevant practitioners and managers who are themselves survivors of domestic abuse, whether disclosed or (very often) undisclosed. Professionals in this situation appear to be part of almost all inter-agency forums, statutory agencies, advocacy groups and domestic violence projects. The fact that they may not have felt able to be open about their status as survivors reinforces the disturbing point we have made throughout, that women continue to be silenced about their experiences of domestic violence. They may be regarded negatively if considered to be still 'in the experience', or speaking from that experience rather than from professional expertise.

Overall, domestic violence survivors have made very significant, often pivotal, contributions to the development both of the women's movement against male violence and of services and policies to protect abused women and to hold perpetrators accountable. Often quietly and without fuss, over the years, women who have suffered abuse themselves have done whatever they can to assist other women in the same situation. Without their work, it is unlikely that policy and practice development would have reached the point it has. We draw this book towards a close by acknowledging this dedicated and often unsung contribution.

Chapter 11

Conclusion

We have described in this book the complex picture which emerged from our research as to the stage reached by user involvement in the domestic violence arena. Looked at from a historical perspective, it was abused women themselves who developed this whole field, both of study and of policy and practice intervention. However, in recent years, most efforts towards change in the domestic violence field have concentrated to a large extent on top-down policy development, while an increased focus on the impact on children and the need to tackle perpetrators has tended to render women 'invisible in their own issue'.

There is a bit of a disjuncture here which this book has attempted to address. Our aim has been to raise survivor voices, and to put them centre stage. To underpin this, we have theorised about the way in which women are typically excluded from conceptualisations of new social movements and abused women service users are rarely seen as a service user group in their own right. Despite the activities of the activist women's movement and the enormous increase in services in recent years, abused women continue to be excluded and overlooked, reinforcing the stigmatisation and silencing that often blight the lives of survivors of violence.

It goes without saying that women's organisations serving the needs of abused women, continue to have the best record of any agencies in listening to service users and in giving them a voice in the wider inter-agency context (although we also identified ways in which they may have retreated to some extent from their previous commitment to the involvement of service users and ex-users in the running and management of services). Both statutory sector agencies and those organisations that have come more recently on to the scene, and for which domestic violence represents only one part of their work, have a substantially poorer record, while inter-agency domestic violence forums represent the meeting-point of both traditions and fall somewhere between the two. The findings of our study have shown that, while almost half of domestic violence inter-agency forums consult service users (as compared to 90 per cent of refuges), there is evidence that many such forums appear to claim that they have a better record at involving women service users than women's refuge and outreach projects in their areas consider they do. Thus, all agencies are closer to 'user involvement' than to 'user control', but multi-agency forums may be underachieving and sometimes, perhaps, over-claiming within this.

Among all agencies, there is more rhetoric than action – intentions are more advanced than practice. Indeed, feedback from women service users themselves suggests that they are relatively unaware of opportunities that do exist to become involved and that often they feel silenced by agencies. Above all, the challenge of enabling abused women to participate in real decision-making, as opposed to possibly cosmetic consultation, has only been met in a handful of locations. The most striking result of this short-fall is the failure of agencies, even after a decade of increasing levels of intervention, to help abused women feel safe in the community – the one thing that survivors have been consistently asking for over all that time, and long before.

More optimistically, there are some examples of best practice in giving a voice to service users and in teasing out common elements that make this work. There is not one, universally applicable, way of doing it. Rather, pioneers are trying out various possibilities and the issue is edging towards becoming expected as standard good practice. Methods being used include the translation of ideas from domestic violence survivors into policy change; the adoption of effective mechanisms for consultation and involvement; and confidence-building and empowerment among survivors themselves on both an individual and a collective level. For user and survivor participation to be an effective and integrated part of service delivery, this book has argued that it needs to be taken seriously and prop-erly resourced (including, for example, the provision possibly of payment or other recompense, and certainly of childcare and expenses, plus support, training, interpreting and access as required). Confidentiality and survivor safety also emerged as vital issues to be considered, as well as representa-tivness and diversity. There needs to be a commitment to translating the results of consultative procedures into action, to reviewing this process and to feeding back the results to those consulted. Without protocols in place to guarantee that consultation and participation are converted into mean-ingful policy and change within the agency or forum concerned, we have argued that it can be pointless to engage in it. Cosmetic exercises are no help to anyone, least of all abuse survivors.

It is important to note that the study found that isolated survivor partici-pation in domestic violence forums, or attendance at forum and other meetings, is generally ineffective (although it can be successful on occa-sion, especially if support is provided). As an alternative, innovative good practice ideas are currently being tried in various parts of the country. These attempts vary from carefully designed consultation strategies (which are hard enough in themselves to put into place and to sustain) to more far-reaching participatory methods and moves towards making services genuinely accountable to service users. At best, abused women are able to have real power in the design and delivery, both of services, and also of participation and consultation exercises themselves. Methods currently being tried include domestic violence survivors' forums or advisory groups feeding into local inter-agency forums, and the active involvement of Women's Aid and of women's support and advocacy projects to represent grass-roots views. Other methods include regular focus groups, questionnaires, user surveys and service evaluations, Internet consultation, Best Value reviews and the use of other existing consultative structures such as Crime and Disorder audits and strategies. An important way forward is for ex-service users and other domestic violence survivors to undertake roles as workers, managers and volunteers, and to participate in the operation of projects. Further, community theatre, poetry workshops and other community arts and campaigns can play a part in influencing policy-makers. All of this can feed into, or be part of, campaigning and activism and the long-nurtured aim of the women's movement to raise abused women's voices.

A vital element of the complexity of the picture – one which perhaps marks out domestic violence work from most other sites of 'user empowerment', and a key proof that power does not operate simplistically in a 'top-down' direction – is that a good number of professionals in relevant statutory and voluntary agencies, and many activists in this field, have themselves been abused. Hence, unlike the field of learning difficulties, for example, there is not the traditionally clear-cut divide between service users and practitioners, between 'us' and 'them'. The study revealed that the presence of abuse survivors in inter-agency and other meetings is currently one of the key ways in which users gain a voice – both directly and indirectly when they speak out themselves or support other women in doing so.

We have referred throughout this book to the role played by such professionals who are themselves survivors of domestic abuse in almost all domestic violence forums and projects. Many have not felt able to be open about their status as survivors, reinforcing the point that women continue to be silenced about their experiences of domestic violence and that they may be regarded negatively if they speak from within that experience rather than solely from professional expertise. It is time to acknowledge and value their contribution, as part of increasing our willingness to respect and listen to survivors of domestic violence. Professionals in this situation have worked tirelessly on behalf of other abused women over many years and service provision has been transformed by their dedicated contributions.

The insights offered in this book are potentially relevant to policy and practice in a range of contexts, and particularly in a climate where government thinking and public expectations increasingly stress consultation and user participation at the local level. It is clear that emancipatory models of exercising accountability to service users in relation to domestic violence can be made a reality, and are worth pursuing, but that they are currently taking considerable effort to achieve. There is a vision here – of services and policy on domestic violence that are truly responsive to abused women's views and are co-ordinated, effective and sensitively informed by their voices. If this can be achieved, domestic violence survivors, policy-makers, service providers and others in society can move forward together towards making the abuse of women a thing of the past. This book is aimed at playing a part in that process and vision.

Epilogue

Words from women survivors of violence

In the Epilogue, we present the words of various women who have experienced domestic violence with whom we spoke during our study, in order to add to the quotations we have used throughout this book. Their words add richness and texture to the arguments, which, under the guidance of the service users and other abuse survivors who have assisted us, we have developed and presented here. We also include a few comments from agency workers.

The epilogue concludes with an account of the innovative Internet project on seeking survivor views that we discussed in Chapter 10. This pioneering consultation was conducted by the Hansard Society and Women's Aid for the All Party Parliamentary Group on Domestic Violence. The account of it presented here has been kindly contributed by the Director of the Women's Aid Federation of England.

Excerpts from an interview with a domestic violence survivor active in policy work

— I have been on all sorts of committees and my experience is that having survivors on a policy committee can be an uneasy situation between everyone. It helps if someone can explain about the power structures and how they work so you can understand them. Then you can understand it better. Otherwise it can be overwhelming ... But, if you can get them to listen properly, then it can be wonderful. The good side is that survivors can then influence policy. Having survivors on the committee can feed in issues about mental health and the effects of domestic violence, or the need for counselling, or the shortfall in services, or whatever it is that is needed.

— But they can be cosmetic – they don't have power, do they.

— I have been on a committee in the past and had no power at all. I felt on my own on this committee. Others are behind my voice, I know, and I felt I had a responsibility to speak for other women, but then I felt so isolated and on my own, I felt I couldn't do it. And that I was being prevented from doing it by the structures.

— But, more recently, I have been listened to more and taken seriously and I feel I have been making a difference. I know I can speak for others now. But if there is a women's group and you are representing that – you would not be so isolated but would be representing the group and others voices more formally. So that can be a help . . . Although, even then, they ignore you if they want to, like I said – even if they pretend they're not doing! They decide behind your back, quietly without telling you, or when you are not there.

— So it takes so long to build it – I do feel that you can do it but it takes a long time to build it up. You have to build it.

— You need the humanness of it.

— And it is about not having any power and not being listened to. And you need to do it on a deep level as human beings, as equals in the endeavour. That's what is so important and is often overlooked by boring procedures and doing it because you feel you have to, not because you are committed to it.

Excerpts from an interview with an agency worker involved in direct work with survivors

— There is a gap between policies and what is happening on the ground. It is wonderful to empower women but not to set them up to fail. And we need more support and resources to avoid this happening. Usually, in my experience, it is hypocrisy. People pretend to listen to survivors' voices and raise everyone's hopes. But usually the agencies are not intending to put energy or resources into actually supporting the women to be part of it or to really take account of what the women say. Not really. So it can be naive or just a smokescreen. It is no good setting it up not to work.

The need for induction, support, self-help and training

This interviewee spoke extensively of the need for training and support in order to conduct advisory work for agencies:

— To do it, you need:

- Self-help – support and warmth between the survivors who are participating so they can help each other as well as doing the agency work.
- Induction and ongoing training – language and structures are alienating to non-professionals. It doesn't have to be like

that, but it is. So survivor representatives need to be trained, 'buddied', supported, offered debriefing or preparation sessions, all that.

- It is very skilled work – it's not easy, it takes a lot of time and care to empower women. And the workers concerned need if possible to have had experience of domestic violence groups and work.

— If you don't provide all this and don't do it properly, you reinforce the stereotypes of what abused women do and think. And the survivors who are put in this position feel a failure, it reinforces our original experience of abuse, so it is doubly victimising. It can be very damaging, feeding into women's feelings that we can't do anything properly. But the only reason why they couldn't do it was in fact because of agency barriers and constraints.

— In some situations, survivors who become trained volunteers can pass on their training to others. Then my view is that they could build up their training portfolios and then perhaps get basic counselling training and get certificates for their portfolios and a certificate in domestic violence awareness training – to build their personal CVs, not just 'help-out'. That's what I tried to do. Survivors often give their time for free so they should get some payback.

— In general, I think it is important:

- To support women into having a voice in a way which is not too huge a transition.
- To make it meaningful.
- To give something back and to be sure you are not merely taking from the women.
- To assist in the setting up of survivors' groups and forums to provide choices and possibilities and autonomy.
- To be more proactive in promoting minority groups (for example, specialist facilities for Asian women's groups).

Excerpts from an interview with a statutory agency worker who is a survivor

— I'll list off some of the issues to be aware of:

- It is important to provide support and confidence-building and training, to treat survivors with respect and equality.
- The wrong personalities can stop it working – you can get some real bust-ups but I suppose that happens everywhere.
- Adequate resources are essential, otherwise you might as well not do it. Providing very small amounts of money can just make it worse.

- It's important to try to reach certain group of survivors and not to only talk to survivors who are motivated to go to meetings and turn up.
- It can be a stepping stone to professionalisation for women and that can be good – get some qualifications and get on in life.
- It is important to keep it going. It's OK as long as more women come and it doesn't become stagnant. You need fresh women all the time. A problem if it is always the same women year after year is that they gradually become more remote from the experience.
- Survivors being consulted don't really represent anyone else.
- It can be a boring and tedious thing to have to keep on doing. Maybe there needs to be more things pulled in – for example, assertiveness training, having fun. To get something out of it. Perhaps women could learn new skills.

— It is vital not to forget the rich and profound contribution of survivors who are professionals, whether or not they talk about it.

Excerpt from an interview with a statutory agency worker who is not a survivor

— While users' perspectives are appreciated in general, this is really a job for professionals, don't you think so?

A selection of individual quotes from different survivors

How things have always been

— Yes, there'd be problems and practical things like looking after children, trying to find a job and somewhere to live. But who'd want us? All of them women are in good jobs, with cars, pensions, nice clothes and there's little old us, no good at anything and the charity shop's best friend. They'd just look down on us! We're nothing, just scum to most people around here. Who cares what we think? Who cares what we feel? We're just out and out losers.
— Nothing changes, people in charge probably don't even listen or read what victims think and just carry on in their own sweet way.
— If there were things concerning survivors (discussed on the domestic violence forum), survivors would be the last to know – there is a gap between forum and survivors – a lack of information, lack of communication.
— We are not neurotic and unstable so don't label us and destroy our self-respect and confidence.

— I think we all get treated the same because that's how people see us – 'The *thems*'.

Beginning to make changes

— Initially I didn't feel I had a right to be there – there were others above my level. I was out of my depth, excluded from networks. I feel better about it now.
— The involvement of survivors could be a ... 'a double-edged sword' – brings up painful memories, but also realising it was not (my) fault, I didn't deserve or cause it. Being involved could bring it all up all the time. But then you wouldn't be alone. It would be easier if it was a long time ago rather than ongoing.
— Women's Aid has the expertise to do it, to consult with survivors and that is helpful because they can do it in a proper way. The disadvantage here is it only reaches some women and it would have to be reorganised, structured, compensated for.
— They are beginning to listen, they are beginning to try. That is a really big thing, isn't it, the fact that they are finally willing to at least *try*.

Difficulties and weaknesses to be overcome

— Women often need support after meetings because they can bring on flashbacks and can be very traumatising. Also meetings are long and boring and they use lots of jargon and are often on about things that, like, you know nothing about. Making grant applications, for example. I mean, how are you expected to know about something like that!?
— I didn't feel part of the meeting even though I was prepared and they tried really hard. They tried so hard! And it was *still* so tedious – all talk, no action. It didn't change anything. The big meetings of the policy people are all talk and the forum was no different – all talk. Talk, talk, talk.
— Why should we do it really? I mean, *really*? Everyone wants to take from us. When I had a burglary in the Lake District they didn't ask me to give advice to the police!
— Why should women disclose it or talk about it? Why *should* they?
— The memories, they hurt, you want to get away from it all. A reminder of bad times, flashbacks, prolonging the misery.
— The shame, embarrassment, stigma – being singled out as 'different' and 'labelled'.
— Safety and confidentiality issues, they are the most important things, plus time to do it.

— It is a good idea but the issues can be too complex for amateur volunteers. Seriously. And I'd hate to see it lead from a good positive thing to being compulsory, like conditional to getting benefits. Like the unemployed now have to go on courses or do voluntary work or lose their benefit. It must *stay* voluntary as it clearly wouldn't appeal to all survivors. After all, who likes meetings? Do *you*?

— Some women find it difficult talking to men, even if it is in an agency.

— Meetings! – What a turn-off!! Ugh. Also, I haven't the time.

— There's a lack of local contact points and meetings. Any get-togethers of women must be easily accessible for volunteers. It is also a trouble if we often move away for housing and lose contact – survivors have to be on the move. You cannot stay in one place so that makes it hard to be involved.

— It could hold you back. It is more important to move on and keep looking ahead, not back over your shoulder to hell on earth.

Good practice

— We do our best on this by listening and encouraging women and paying expenses. Finding a time, a date and venue to suit a group of women is very, very difficult, especially as professional workers only want daytime meetings, which isn't always easy for women, but neither are evenings unless they own a car. It's tough to get it right. (Interview with professional who is also a survivor.)

— Practical help – transport, crèche, childcare, expenses; an advisory or attendance fee you get for doing it – but you would need to ensure women went along for the right reasons, not just for the cash; letting women know it is happening and being actually invited to participate! Otherwise, how do you get there? Also, a 'sitting-in' type of apprenticeship. Maybe go with a refuge worker, or another worker until you know the ropes. It's a bit overwhelming to think about doing it, though! Not on your own.

— You go and you're learning more about meetings and how to behave there before you actually go and that helps.

— Yes, they have to take on equalities issues, of course they do. Like racism, like you said. Sexuality – I wondered when you'd ask. I bet you assumed I was in a heterosexual relationship.

— When it works, it helps you overcome things – hear other people's experiences. Learn to stay away from situations that could lead to trouble. Speaking out helps yourself and others – gives you confidence.

— The way it helps is by making them know what it's *really* like and what help you need at the time. They learn what women really want and can tell others. It gives back a bit of power.

— The women act as a check and monitor on any proposed changes in services. Also as advisors, putting forward their ideas. It's great, and the agencies really do listen now. (Interview with professional who is also a survivor.)

— We are there as a right and have equal say with anyone else. We can raise any issues and will always be listened to. For example, the forum took up the anti-discrimination and 'no men' policies from survivors' comments and the need for a helpline came from women and is being actually done now.

— Being involved in agencies uses women's own experience. What happened to you is actually important. It can be therapeutic for women – a chance to meet and share with others who know what domestic violence is like. Learn you are not alone.

— Survivor representation – they still haven't got it right on involvement of survivors, have they? But it can help to co-ordinate and improve local provision, so it's bound to be good for survivors. I've seen it help in practice. Although it can be intimidating unless you are a strong woman like me.

— For women who have experienced violence to meet, you need:

  • To be listened to, to have a voice.
  • Transport and a crèche or other childcare and expenses.
  • Practical help with doing it.
  • More advertisements.
  • Support and confidence-building in public speaking.
  • A slot reserved in the meeting for survivors only to speak.
  • Training, leading on to paid work.
  • To make it interesting and fun, not boring.
  • More invitations to join in from the agencies.
  • Suitable times and places for meetings.
  • Anonymous places to meet, not in buildings with 'domestic violence' plastered all over doors!
  • Shorter meetings – seriously!'

(From a group interview with survivors who have been active in policy work.)

Women's needs

— Some women need social services but the main needs are for the police to take it seriously and act quickly, and for housing and benefits to be available so you've got somewhere to go and some money to do it.

— We need prompt action and to be listened to, and for the services to be available, not cut back all the time. What we need is a lot more refuges. Services are still so inadequate.

— You need early intervention. Shouting and threatening and being restricted is devastating. And it always gets worse – a crescendo. Getting out early is what you need. Mother and toddler groups could discuss it and the effects on children – discuss it in all sorts of places, so women know what to do.

Improvements survivors would like to see (summarised from various interviews)

- The employment of more survivors in agencies concerned with domestic violence.
- More information, more 24-hour helplines, more information on TV.
- More information for abused women in the community (rather than only available in refuges).
- Outreach projects.
- More support for women who have left a refuge and been rehoused.
- Advocates who can be a bridge between women and different agencies.
- Members of staff specialising in domestic violence in agencies like the Benefits Agency.
- Asking women if they would like to become involved in domestic violence forums on exit questionnaires; asking women what they think.
- More severe penalties for perpetrators.
- Fewer delays in bringing cases to court.
- Teaching schoolchildren about domestic violence.
- More resources for domestic violence and an end to pushing two-parent, two-children families.

A group of survivors made the following list of general improvements they would like to see:

- More awareness.
- Better posters.
- To be believed.
- To be listened to.
- Language difficulties and cultural issues taken on.
- More training and understanding from police.
- A more reliable service from the police.
- More safety and security.
- Confidentiality.
- Refuges and outreach – more of them.

- More support groups.
- More helplines and one stop shops.
- Publicity in supermarkets, TV and so on.
- Making sure no workers overlook safety issues.
- Speedy responses which are proactive and safe.
- Services which improve things for children who get dragged around to all the interviews and agencies.
- Making women and children safer.
- Making services more responsive.

Issues for Women's Aid

— Women have the right in Women's Aid, yes, but Women's Aid doesn't do that so much now as it used to. You still have it but ... Now it's all policies and management and protocols and not much time for the women. Refuges tend to have a full-time manager who never works with the women, so it's not much of a collective any more. They've forgotten about empowerment a bit. (Interview with Women's Aid worker who is a survivor.)

— The old policy of trying to offer jobs to suitable ex-residents in Women's Aid was great. Women's Aid don't do that so much now. Now you need qualifications and to be good on computers. It's not so hands on any more.

— Yes, Women's Aid is great. Women are there automatically, as a right. You just feel that you are important and they will listen to you.

— It would be good if refuges could talk to women and then pass on what we think. If it was done properly. But refuge workers don't have time to do it. They don't even have time to go to meetings – how could they consult with women as well? They need time and resources if they are to do that. The other agencies need to realise.

A final word

One woman ended a general discussion of survivor participation by saying:

Do you know what made it really good? Knowing change was a real possibility. Being actively sought out as survivors. Encouraged and made to feel we were valued and listened to. It's a problem when nothing happens about things women suggest – they feel ignored and may not know about all the practical real reasons why services are slow to change. So women need training and encouragement, assertive training, that sort of thing. The policy people need to reach out to women in domestic violence situations because they feel isolated and see no way out. Help to make them more positive.

Womenspeak

A parliamentary Internet consultation with domestic violence survivors

Nicola Harwin CBE, Director, Women's Aid Federation of England

In 1999, the All Party Parliamentary Group on Domestic Violence was formed as a cross-party network of MPs and peers who were concerned about violence against women. This Group worked in partnership with the Hansard Society and with Women's Aid in March 2000 to conduct the first ever on-line consultation with survivors of domestic violence. The aim was to offer an opportunity for survivors of domestic violence to share their experiences and concerns directly with parliamentarians through the Internet, and for this to inform parliamentarians in their work to develop appropriate laws and policy.

The project was an innovative consultation, using new interactive technology, with the aim of enabling socially excluded citizens to input their views and concerns into a parliamentary debate. It was also part of a new movement for pushing forward the progress of e-democracy in the UK, and set an example for more widespread e-consultation, citizen involvement and feedback as part of the political process at national and local level.

For some of the women who participated, the potential of information technology was opened up for the first time. Prior to the month-long consultation, the project co-ordinator, based at the Hansard Society, worked with national staff from the Women's Aid Federation of England and with local Women's Aid refuge organisations for several months to plan and promote the process. Complicated, but necessary, systems were established to enable password access to the site but also to ensure anonymity and safety. Local resources for Internet access were set up, and provision for personal support for participants from refuge services, outreach services and the wider community was established.

Throughout one month, MPs from the All Party Group also encouraged local organisations to join in the debate and to contribute individually. In Luton, the constituency of Margaret Moran MP, Chair of the All Party Parliamentary Group on Domestic Violence, the first women to log on were a group of Irish women travellers, many of whom could not read or write, but who, with assistance, were able to contribute their own experiences and their views on government policy towards domestic violence. In some areas, local community centres were made available for survivors who wished to use the Web for free, and assistance was organised for those who had never used the Internet before.

Hearing the direct experiences of women survivors is a powerful tool in making informed decisions on domestic violence. There were almost a thousand contributions to the site from women who have lived with domestic violence during the course of the month-long consultation. Many women discussed their experiences for the first time, secure in the anonymity that on-line discussion provides. Many contributors simply sought help and found this easy using the link to the Women's Aid website, the Women's Aid National Domestic Violence Helpline and the UK-wide network of local refuge services. There was a strong call for the site to be continued as a forum for support and discussion and for consultation on best practice. (The *i-village exploring abuse* website was set up subsequently and helped meet some of that need.)

The results of the consultation showed clearly that there was a very piecemeal response to domestic violence by many agencies across the country and that there was a lack of common standards for good practice. Survivors were also asked to contribute to a wish list of 'What women want', a summary of the results of which are reproduced below. Since the consultation, the results and the evidence that it provided about the problems still faced by women and children experiencing domestic violence, as well as their recommendations for change, have been used to take forward the work programme of the Parliamentary Group and of relevant agencies.

Women's Aid, which provides secretariat support to the All Party Group on Domestic Violence, has worked with the Group to evaluate the findings and wish list against the measures identified in the government report *Living Without Fear* (Cabinet Office, 1999), and also against the recommendations set out in *Families Without Fear*, the Women's Aid National Agenda for Action (Women's Aid Federation of England, 1998). This has helped to identify areas of policy and practice where more rapid progress needs to be made.

In particular, the work of the All Party Group since 2000 has focused on three key areas identified by survivors:

- The need for changes to the Children Act 1989 – reflecting concerns about the safety of women and children in child contact arrangements with violent fathers.
- Policy and practice relating to immigration law and forced marriages.
- The impact of proposals in Supporting People on the funding of essential refuge and outreach services.

Many of the findings of the Womenspeak consultation with survivors confirmed the evidence from research and from Women's Aid, building on work with survivors over the past thirty years. They have also been reconfirmed by subsequent research into survivors' experiences, *Routes to Safety*, which was commissioned by Women's Aid and recently published (Humphreys and Thiara, 2002).

The stories of abused women, which were included in the Womenspeak report, highlight how they had faced difficulties, often in relation to ongoing problems that lasted many years. The consultation demonstrated clearly how domestic violence is not a one-off event and how it is not something that only occurs when relationships split up, but, rather, is part of a pattern of ongoing controlling behaviour, which can be life-threatening and which can affect all aspects of the lives of abused women and their children. The findings clearly point to the need for proactive responses by all agencies to name the problem and to take responsibility for providing an effective response to protect the safety and rights of survivors.

It is now two years since Womenspeak, and it is heartening to note that there has been more progress in developing effective responses by national government and by some statutory agencies in that time. In particular, there has been significant progress in criminal justice responses and, at the time of writing, new proposals for legislative change. Nevertheless, the voices of many of those survivors who contributed to Womenspeak are still waiting to be heard, and their wish list is still as relevant and current as it was in March 2000.

Summary of Womenspeak findings

What women want

- Positive action by all agencies.
- More resources for refuge and outreach services.
- Equal support for women from minority groups and help for all abused women regardless of immigration status.
- More publicity and information.
- Domestic violence to be treated as a crime, and better protection.
- Mandatory training of legal professionals and courts to prioritise the safety of the survivor.
- Changes to child contact law and protection from post-separation violence.
- More specialist services for children to help deal with their experiences.
- More flexible housing options.
- Better legal protection to help women stay safe in their own homes.
- Help to protect possessions and pets if they have to leave.
- Access to benefits and economic independence, e.g. fast track benefits system in an emergency; better access to Social Fund payments; training opportunities; storage for existing possessions.

Bibliography

Abrahams, C. (1994) *The Hidden Victims: Children and domestic violence*, London: NCH Action for Children.

Abrahams, H. (forthcoming) 'A long hard road to go by: A study of support needs in Women's Aid refuges', unpublished Ph.D. thesis, University of Bristol.

Adams, R. (1996) *Social Work and Empowerment*, Basingstoke: Macmillan.

Anderson, J. (1996) 'Yes, but IS IT empowerment? Initiation, implementation and outcomes of community action', in Humphries, B. (ed.) *Critical Perspectives on Empowerment*, Birmingham: Venture Press.

Aris, R., Hague, G. and Mullender, A. (2003) 'Defined by men's abuse: the "spoiled identity" of domestic violence survivors', in Stanko, E. A. (ed.) *The Meanings of Violence*, London: Routledge.

Baistow, K. (1994) 'Liberation and regulation? Some paradoxes of empowerment', *Critical Social Policy* 42: 34–46.

Barker, I. and Peck, E. (1987) *Power in Strange Places: User empowerment in mental health services*, London: Good Practices in Mental Health.

Barnes, M. (1997) *Care, Communities and Citizens*, Harlow: Addison Wesley Longman.

Barnes, M. (1999) 'Users as citizens: collective action and the local governance of welfare', *Social Policy and Administration* 33(1): 73–90.

Barnes, M. and Bowl, R. (2001) *Taking Over the Asylum: Empowerment and mental health*, Basingstoke: Palgrave.

Barnes, M., Harrison, S., Mort, M. and Shardlow, P. (1999) *Unequal Partners: User groups and community care*, Bristol: The Policy Press.

Barnes, M., Harrison, S., Mort, M., Shardlow, P. and Wistow, G. (1996) *Consumerism and Citizenship among Users of Health and Care Services*, End of Award Report to the ESRC (Award No. L311253025), Birmingham: University of Birmingham.

Barnes, M. and Oliver, M. (1995) 'Disability rights: rhetoric and reality in the UK', *Disability and Society* 10(1): 111–16.

Barnes, M. and Warren, L. (eds) (1999) *Paths to Empowerment*, Bristol: The Policy Press.

Batsleer, J. and Humphries, B. (eds) (2000) *Welfare, Exclusion and Political Agency*, London: Routledge.

Batsleer, J., Burman, E., Chantler, K., McIntosh, H., Pantling, K., Smailes, S. and Warner, S. (2002) *Domestic Violence and Minoritisation: Supporting women to independence*, Manchester: Manchester Metropolitan University.

Baumgartner, F. and Leech, B. (1998) *Basic Interests: The importance of groups in politics and political science*, Princeton, NJ: Princeton University Press.

Begum, N. (1992) 'Disabled women and the feminist agenda', in Hinds, H., Phoenix, A. and Stacey, J. (eds) *Working Out: New directions for women's studies*, London: Falmer.

Bennett, G. and Kingston, P. (1993) *Elder Abuse: Concepts, theories and interventions*, London: Chapman and Hall.

Beresford, P. (1997) 'Towards an empowering social work practice: learning from service users and their movements', in *Empowerment Practice in Social Work: Developing richer conceptual foundations*. Conference Papers, 24–6 September 1997, Toronto: University of Toronto, Faculty of Social Work.

Beresford, P. (2001) 'Service users, social policy and the future of welfare', *Critical Social Policy* 21(4): 494–512.

Beresford, P. and Campbell, J. (1994) 'Disabled people, service users, user involvement and representation', *Disability and Society* 9(3): 315–25.

Beresford, P. and Croft, S. (1995) 'It's our problem too! Challenging the exclusion of the poor people from poverty decisions', *Critical Social Policy* 44/5.

Beresford, P. and Croft, S. (2001) 'Service users' knowledges and the social construction of social work', *Journal of Social Work* 1(3): 295–316.

Binney, V., Harknell, G. and Nixon, J. (1981) *Leaving Violent Men: A study of refuges and housing for abused women*, Leeds: Women's Aid Federation of England.

Bossey, J. and Coleman, S. (2000) *Womenspeak: Findings of the parliamentary domestic violence Internet consultation*, Bristol: Women's Aid Federation of England.

Boushell, M. (1994) 'The protective environment of children: towards a framework for anti-oppressive, cross-cultural and cross-national understanding', *British Journal of Social Work* 24: 173–90.

Brandon, D. (1991) *Innovation Without Change: Consumer control of psychiatric services*, London: Macmillan.

Braye, S. (2000) 'Participation and involvement in social care: an overview', in Kemshall, H. and Littlechild, R. (eds) *User Involvement and Participation in Social Care: Research informing practice*, London: Jessica Kingsley, pp. 142–3.

Brent Asian Women's Resource Centre (2000–1) *Asian Women's Resource Centre: Twenty-one years of providing for her, for you, for a better community*, Brent: Asian Women's Resource Centre.

Bridge Child Care Consultancy Service (1991) *Sukina: An evaluation of the circumstances leading to her death*, London: Bridge Child Care Consultancy Service.

Cabinet Office (1999) *Living Without Fear*, London: Women's Unit of the Cabinet Office.

Campbell, J. and Oliver, M. (1996) *Disability Politics: Understanding our past, changing our future*, London: Routledge.

Campbell, P. (1996) 'The history of the user movement in the United Kingdom', in Heller, T., Reynolds, J., Gomm, R., Muston, R. and Pattison, S. (eds) *Mental Health Matters*, Basingstoke: Macmillan.

Chamberlin, J. (1988) *On Our Own: Patient-controlled alternatives to the mental health system*, London: MIND.

Charles, N. (2000) *Feminism, the State and Social Policy*, Basingstoke: Macmillan.

Cheshire Domestic Abuse Project (2002) *Qualitative Survey of Women's Aid Service Users* (unpublished).

Cooper, L., Coote, A., Davies, A. and Jackson, C. (1995) *Voices Off: Tackling the democratic deficit in health*, London: Institute for Public Policy Research.

Coote, A. and Campbell, B. (1987) *Sweet Freedom: The struggle for women's liberation*, 2nd edn, Oxford: Basil Blackwell.

Croft, S. and Beresford, P. (1996) 'The politics of participation', in Taylor, D. (ed.) *Critical Social Policy: A reader*, London: Sage. (Originally published in *Critical Social Policy* 35(Autumn): 20–44.)

Croft, S. and Beresford, P. (2002) 'Service users' perspectives', in Davies, M. (ed.) *The Blackwell Companion to Social Work*, 2nd edn, Oxford: Blackwell.

Cross, M. (1999) 'Review of domestic violence and child abuse: policy and practice issues for local authorities and other agencies', in Greater London Action on Disability (eds) *Boadicea*, London: Greater London Action on Disability.

Cull, L. and Roche, J. (eds) (2001) *The Law and Social Work*, Buckingham: Open University Press.

Dalton, R. J. and Kuechler, M. (1990) *Challenging the Political Order: New social and political movements in Western democracies*, Oxford: Oxford University Press.

Davies, M. (1994) *Women and Violence: Realities and responses worldwide*, London: Zed Books.

Davis, K. (1994) 'What's in a voice? Methods and metaphors', in *Feminism and Psychology* 4(3): 353–61.

Department of Health (1996a) *Community Service Users as Consultants and Trainers*, Leeds: The NHS Executive Community Care Branch. (Produced by Vivien Lindow on behalf of the National User Involvement Evaluation Group.)

Department of Health (1996b) *Encouraging User Involvement in Commissioning: A resource for commissioners*, Leeds: The NHS Executive Community Care Branch. (Produced by Jenny Morris on behalf of the National User Involvement Evaluation Group.)

Department of Health (2000) *Domestic Violence: A resource manual for health care professionals*, London: Department of Health.

Department of Health (2001) *Valuing People: A new strategy for learning disability for the 21st century*, London: The Stationery Office.

DETR (Department of the Environment, Transport and the Regions), Department of Health, Department of Social Security, HM Treasury, Home Office, Scottish Office, Welsh Office and Women's Unit (1998) *Supporting People: A new policy and funding framework for support services*, London: Department of Social Security.

Dobash, R. E. and Dobash, R. P. (1980) *Violence Against Wives: A case against the patriarchy*, Shepton Mallet: Open Books.

Dobash, R. E. and Dobash, R. P. (1992) *Women, Violence and Social Change*, London and New York: Routledge.

Dobash, R. E., Dobash, R. P. and Cavanagh, K. (1985) 'The contact between battered women and social and medical agencies', in Pahl, J. (ed.) *Private Violence and Public Policy*, London: Routledge.

Dobash, R. P. and Dobash, R. E. (1981) 'Community responses to violence against wives: charivari, abstract justice and patriarchy', *Social Problems* 28(5): 563–81.

Dobash, R. P., Dobash, R. E., Cavanagh, K. and Lewis, R. (2000) *Changing Violent Men*, London: Sage.

Dominy, N. and Radford, L. (1996) *Domestic Violence in Surrey: Developing an effective inter-agency response*, Guildford: Surrey County Council/Roehampton Institute.

Dowson, S. (1997) 'Empowerment within services: a comfortable delusion', in Ramcharan, P., Roberts, G., Grant, G. and Borland, J. (eds) *Empowerment in Everyday Life: Learning disability*, London: Jessica Kingsley.

Dullea, K. and Mullender, A. (1999) 'Evaluation and empowerment', in Shaw, I. and Lishman, J. (eds) *Evaluation and Social Work Practice*, London: Sage.

Edwards, R. and Ribbens, J. (1998) 'Living on the edges: public knowledge, private lives, personal experience', in Ribbens, J. and Edwards, R. (eds) *Feminist Dilemmas in Qualitative Research*, London: Sage.

Edwards, S. (2001) 'New directions in prosecution', in Taylor-Browne, J. (ed.) *What Works in Reducing Domestic Violence? A comprehensive guide for professionals*, London: Whiting and Birch.

Eschle, C. (2001) *Global Democracy, Social Movements and Feminism*, Boulder, CO: West View Press.

ESRC Violence Research Programme (1998) *Taking Stock: What do we know about violence?*, Uxbridge: Brunel University, ESRC Violence Research Programme.

Figueira-McDonough, J. (1998) 'Toward a gender-integrated knowledge in social work', in Figueira-McDonough, J., Netting, F. E. and Nichols-Casebolt, A. (eds) *The Role of Gender in Practice Knowledge: Claiming half the human experience*, New York and London: Garland Publishing.

Forbes, J. and Sashidharan, S. (1997) 'User involvement in services: incorporation or challenge?', *British Journal of Social Work* 27(4): 481–98.

Foucault, M. (1979) *The History of Sexuality, Vol. 1: An introduction*, trans. Robert Hurley, London: Allen Lane.

Freeman, J. (1972–3) 'The tyranny of structurelessness', *Berkeley Journal of Sociology* 17: 151–64.

Freeman, M. (1979) *Violence in the Home*, Farnborough: Saxon House.

Gelb, J. (1990) 'Feminism and political action', in Dalton, R. J. and Kuechler, M. (eds) *Challenging the Political Order: New social and political movements in Western democracies*, Oxford: Oxford University Press.

Gillman, M. (1996) 'Empowering professionals in higher education', in Humphries, B. (ed.) *Critical Perspectives on Empowerment*, Birmingham: Venture Press.

Goffman, E. (1963) *Stigma: Notes on the management of spoiled identity*, Englewood Cliffs, NJ: Prentice-Hall.

Gondolf, E. (1998) 'Multi-site evaluation of batterer intervention systems: reliability and validity of outcome measures for batterer intervention evaluation'. Online. Available at www.mincava.umn.edu/arts/asp.

Grace, S. (1995) *Policing Domestic Violence in the 1990s*, HORS Report No. 139, London: Home Office.

Grant, G. (1997) 'Consulting to involve or consulting to empower?', in Ramcharan, P., Roberts, G., Grant, G. and Borland, J. (eds) *Empowerment in Everyday Life: Learning disability*, London: Jessica Kingsley.

Grant, W. (2000) *Pressure Groups and British Politics*, Basingstoke: Palgrave.

Grant, W. (2002) 'Direct action, when it works, may stifle political action', *The Times Higher Education Supplement*, 19 April: 20–1.

Greenbaum, T. (2000) *Moderating Focus Groups: A practical guide for group facilitation*, 2nd edn, London: Sage.

Greenwich Asian Women's Project (1995) *Asian Women and Domestic Violence: Information for advisers*, London: London Borough of Greenwich.

Grotberg, E. (1997) 'The International Resilience Project', in John, M. (ed.) *A Charge Against Society: The child's right to protection*, London: Jessica Kingsley.

Hague, G. (2000) 'What works? Multi-agency initiatives', in Home Office (eds) *Reducing Domestic Violence: What works?*, Briefing Notes, London: Home Office.

Hague, G. (2001) 'What works in reducing domestic violence: multi-agency initiatives', in Taylor Browne, J. (ed.) *What Works in Reducing Domestic Violence? A comprehensive guide for professionals*, London: Whiting and Birch.

Hague, G. (2002) *Domestic Violence in Brent: Needs, strengths and gaps: An assessment of domestic violence services*, London Borough of Brent: Community Safety Team.

Hague, G. and Malos, E. (1998) *Domestic Violence: Action for change*, 2nd edn, Cheltenham: New Clarion Press.

Hague, G. and Wilson, C. (1996) *The Silenced Pain*, Bristol: The Policy Press.

Hague, G. and Wilson, C. (2000) 'The silenced pain', *Journal of Gender Studies* 9(2): 157–65.

Hague, G., Malos, E. and Dear, W. (1996) *Multi-agency Work and Domestic Violence*, Bristol: The Policy Press.

Hague, G., Kelly, L., Malos, E., Mullender, A. and Debbonaire, T. (1996a) *Children, Domestic Violence and Refuges: A study of needs and responses*, Bristol: Women's Aid Federation of England.

Hague, G., Mullender, A., Aris, R. and Dear, W. (2001) *Abused Women's Perspectives*, End of Award Report to the ESRC (Award No. L133251017), Bristol: University of Bristol.

Hague, G., Kelly, L. and Mullender, A. (2001a) *Challenging Violence Against Women: The Canadian experience*, Bristol: The Policy Press.

Hague, G., Mullender, A. and Aris, R. (2002) *Professionals by Experience: A guide to service user participation and consultation for domestic violence services*, Bristol: Women's Aid Federation of England.

Hanmer, J., Itzen, K., with Quaid, S. and Wigglesworth, D. (eds) (2000) *Home Truths about Domestic Violence: Feminist influences on policy and practice*, London: Routledge.

Harding, S. (1993) 'Rethinking standpoint epistemology', in Alcoff, A. and Potter, E. (eds) *Feminist Epistemologies*, London: Routledge.

Harding, T. and Beresford, P. (1996) *The Standards We Expect: What service users and carers want from social services workers*, London: National Institute for Social Work.

Harding, T. and Oldman, H. (1996) *Involving Service Users and Carers in Local Services*, London: National Institute for Social Work; Thames Ditton: Surrey Social Services Department.

Harwin, N. (1999) 'New opportunities, old challenges: a perspective from Women's Aid', in Harwin, N., Hague, G. and Malos, E. (eds) *The Multi-agency Approach to Domestic Violence: New opportunities, old challenges?*, London: Whiting and Birch.

Harwin, N., Malos, E. and Hague, G. (eds) (1999) *The Multi-agency Approach to Domestic Violence: New opportunities, old challenges*, London: Whiting and Birch.

Hastings, A., McArthur, A. and McGregor, A. (1996) *Less than Equal: Community organisations and estate regeneration*, Bristol: The Policy Press.

Healy, K. (2000) *Social Work Practices: Contemporary perspectives on change*, London: Sage.

Hen Co-op (1993) *Growing Old Disgracefully*, London: Piatkus.

Hen Co-op (1995) *Disgracefully Yours*, London: Piatkus.

Henderson, S. (1997) *Service Provision for Women Experiencing Domestic Violence in Scotland*, Edinburgh: Scottish Office Central Research Unit.

Hester, M. and Pearson, C. (1998) *From Periphery to Centre: Domestic violence in work with abused children*, Bristol: The Policy Press.

Hester, M., Pearson, C. and Harwin, N. (2000) *Making an Impact: A reader*, London: Jessica Kingsley.

Hill Collins, P. (1991) *Black Feminist Thought: Knowledge, consciousness and the politics of empowerment*, New York: Routledge.

Hoff, L. A. (1990) *Battered Women as Survivors*, London and New York: Routledge.

Home Office (1990) *Circular 60/90: Domestic violence*, London: HMSO.

Home Office (1991) *The Citizen's Charter*, London: HMSO.

Home Office (1995) *Inter-agency Circular: Inter-agency coordination to tackle domestic violence*, London: Home Office.

Home Office (1999) *Multi-agency Guidance for Addressing Domestic Violence*, London: HMSO.

Home Office (2000) *Reducing Domestic Violence: What works?*, Briefing Notes, London: HMSO.

Home Office (2000a) *Domestic Violence: Revised circular to the police*, London: Home Office, Policing and Crime Reduction Group.

Homer, N., Leonard, A., and Taylor, P. (1984) *Private Violence, Public Shame: A report on the circumstances of women leaving refuges*, Middlesborough: Cleveland Refuge and Aid for Women and Children.

Humphreys, C. (2000) *Social Work, Domestic Violence and Child Protection: Challenging practice*, Bristol: The Policy Press.

Humphreys, C. and Mullender, A. (2002) *Children and Domestic Violence*, Dartington: Department of Health Unit.

Humphreys, C. and Thiara, R. (2002) *Routes to Safety: Protection issues facing abused women and children and the role of outreach services*, Bristol: Women's Aid Federation of England.

Humphreys, C., Hester, M., Hague, G., Mullender, A., Abrahams, H. and Lowe, P. (2000) *From Good Intentions to Good Practice: Mapping services working with families where there is domestic violence*, Bristol: The Policy Press.

Humphries, B. (ed.) (1996) *Critical Perspectives on Empowerment*, Birmingham: Venture Press.

James-Hanman, D. (1994) *Domestic Violence: Help, advice and information for disabled women*, London: London Borough of Hounslow.

James-Hanman, D. (1995) *The Needs and Experiences of Black and Minority Ethnic Women Experiencing Domestic Violence*, London: London Borough of Islington Women's Equality Unit.

James-Hanman, D. (2000) 'Enhancing multi-agency work', in Hanmer, J., Itzen, K., Quaid, S. and Wigglesworth, D. (eds) (2000) *Home Truths about Domestic Violence: Feminist influences on policy and practice*, London: Routledge.

Kelly, L. (1988) 'How women define their experiences of violence', in Yllo, K. and Bograd, M. (eds) *Feminist Perspectives on Wife Abuse*, London: Sage.

Kelly, L. (1999) *Domestic Violence Matters: An evaluation of a development project*, Home Office Research Study 193, London: Home Office.

Kelly, L. and Humphreys, C. (2000) 'What works in reducing domestic violence? Outreach and advocacy approaches', in Home Office (eds) *Reducing Domestic Violence: What works?*, Briefing Notes, London: Home Office.

Kelly, L. and Humphreys, C. (2001) 'Supporting women and children in their communities: outreach and advocacy approaches to domestic violence', in Taylor-Browne, J. (ed.) *What Works in Reducing Domestic Violence? A comprehensive guide for professionals*, London: Whiting and Birch.

Kelly, L., Burton, S. and Regan, L. (1996) 'Beyond victim or survivor: sexual violence, identity and feminist theory and practice', in Adkins, L. and Merchant, V. (eds) *Sexualizing the Social: Power and the organization of sexuality*, Basingstoke: Macmillan.

Kirkwood, C. (1993) *Leaving Abusive Partners: From the scars of survival to the wisdom for change*, London: Sage.

Krueger, R. (2000) *Focus Groups: A practical guide for applied research*, 3rd edn, London: Sage.

Law Commission (1995) *Mental Incapacity*, London: HMSO.

Leonard, P. (1997) *Postmodern Welfare: Reconstructing an emancipatory project*, London: Sage.

Lindow, V. (1994) *Self-help Alternatives to Mental Health Services*, London: MIND.

Lindow, V. (1994a) *Purchasing Mental Health Services: Self-help alternatives*, London: MIND.

Lindow, V. (1995) *Service User Involvement: Synthesis of findings and experience in the field*, York: York Publishing Services.

London Borough of Lewisham's Community Safety Team in conjunction with the Lewisham Domestic Violence Forum (1998) *Survey of Domestic Violence Services in Lewisham*, London: London Borough of Lewisham.

Lovenduski, J. (1993) *Contemporary Feminist Politics: Women and power in Britain*, Oxford: Oxford University Press.

Lukes, S. (1974) *Power: A radical view*, London: Macmillan.

Malos, E. and Hague, G. (1993) *Domestic Violence and Housing: Local authority responses to women and children escaping violence in the home*, Bristol: Women's Aid Federation of England and University of Bristol.

Mama, A. (1996) *The Hidden Struggle: Statutory and voluntary sector responses to violence against black women in the home*, London: Whiting and Birch. (First published in 1989.)

Maynard, M. (1985) 'The response of social workers to domestic violence', in Pahl, J. (ed.) *Private Violence and Public Policy: The needs of battered women and the response of the public services*, London: Routledge and Kegan Paul.

Maynard, M. and Purvis, J. (eds) (1994) *Researching Women's Lives from a Feminist Perspective*, London: Taylor and Francis.

McGee, C. (2000) *Childhood Experiences of Domestic Violence*, London: Jessica Kingsley.

McIntosh, M. (1996) 'Feminism and social policy', in Taylor, D. (ed.) *Critical Social Policy: A reader*, London: Sage.

McWilliams, M. and McKiernan, J. (1993) *Bringing It Out in the Open: Domestic violence services in Northern Ireland*, Belfast: HMSO.

Means, R., and Smith, R. (1996) *Community Care and Homelessness: Living with domestic violence*, London: Whiting and Birch.

Members of Women First (2002) 'Women First: A self-directed group for women with and without learning disabilities – our experiences 1990–99', in Cohen, M. B. and Mullender, A. (eds) *Gender and Groupwork*, London: Routledge.

Mirrlees-Black, C. (1999) *Domestic Violence: Findings from a new British crime survey self-completion questionnaire*, Home Office Research Study 191, London: Home Office.

Mooney, J. (1994) *The Hidden Figure: Domestic violence in North London*, London: Middlesex University.

Mooney, J. (2000) *Gender, Violence and the Social Order*, Basingstoke: Macmillan.

Morley, R. (2000) 'Domestic violence and housing', in Hanmer, J., Itzen, K., Quaid, S. and Wigglesworth, D. (eds) *Home Truths about Domestic Violence: Feminist influences on policy and practice*, London: Routledge.

Morris, J. (1991) *Pride Against Prejudice: Transforming attitudes to disability*, London: The Women's Press.

Morris, J. (1994) *The Shape of Things to Come? User-led social services*, Social Services Policy Forum Paper No. 3, London: National Institute of Social Work.

Morris, J. (ed.) (1996) *Encounters with Strangers: Feminism and disability*, London: The Women's Press.

Mullender, A. (1995) 'Review article: towards mental health for women', *Issues in Social Work Education* 15(2): 81–9.

Mullender, A. (1996) *Rethinking Domestic Violence: The social work and probation response*, London: Routledge.

Mullender, A. and Burton, S. (2000) 'What works in reducing domestic violence: perpetrator programmes', in Home Office (eds) *Reducing Domestic Violence: What works?*, Briefing Notes, London: Home Office.

Mullender, A. and Burton, S. (2001) 'Dealing with perpetrators', in Taylor-Browne, J. (ed.) *What Works in Reducing Domestic Violence? A comprehensive guide for professionals*, London: Whiting and Birch.

Mullender, A. and Hague, G. (2000) 'What works in reducing domestic violence: women survivors' views', in Home Office (eds) *Reducing Domestic Violence: What works?*, Briefing Notes, London: Home Office.

Mullender, A. and Hague, G. (2001) 'Reducing domestic violence: what works? Women survivors' views', in Taylor-Browne, J. (ed.) *What Works in Reducing Domestic Violence? A comprehensive guide for professionals*, London: Whiting and Birch.

Mullender, A. and Morley, R. (1994) *Children Living with Domestic Violence: Putting men's abuse of women on the child care agenda*, London: Whiting and Birch.

Mullender, A. and Ward, D. (1991) *Self-directed Groupwork: Users take action for empowerment*, London: Whiting and Birch.

Mullender, A., Kelly, L., Hague, G., Malos, E. and Imam, U. (2000) *Children's Needs, Coping Strategies and Understandings of Woman Abuse*, End of Award

Report to the ESRC (Award No. L129251037), Coventry: University of Warwick, Department of Social Policy and Social Work.

Mullender, A., Hague, G., Imam, U., Kelly, L., Malos, E. and Regan, L. (2002) *Children's Perspectives on Domestic Violence*, London: Sage.

O'Hagan, M. (1993) *Stopovers on My Way Home from Mars: A journey into the psychiatric survivor movement in the USA, Britain and the Netherlands*, London: Survivors Speak Out.

Okun, L. (1986) *Woman Abuse: Facts replacing myths*, Albany, NY: State University of New York Press.

Oliver, M. (1990) *The Politics of Disablement*, Basingstoke: Macmillan.

Pahl, J. (1985) *Private Violence and Public Policy: The needs of battered women and the residents of refuges*, London: Routledge and Kegan Paul.

Park, Y., Fedler, J. and Dangor, Z. (2000) *Reclaiming Women's Spaces: New perspectives on violence against women and sheltering in South Africa*, Lenasia, SA: Nisaa.

Pease, B. (2002) 'Rethinking empowerment: a postmodern reappraisal for emancipatory practice', *British Journal of Social Work* 32(2): 135–47.

Pease, B. and Fook, J. (eds) (1999) *Transforming Social Work Practice: Postmodern critical perspectives*, London: Routledge.

Pence, E. and Shephard, M. (eds) (1999) *The Co-ordinated Community Response: The Duluth experience*, London: Sage.

Pleck, E. (1986) *Domestic Tyranny: The making of American social policy against family violence from colonial times to the present*, Oxford: Oxford University Press.

Plotnikoff, J. and Woolfson, R. (1998) *Policing Domestic Violence: Effective organisational structures*. Police Research Series Paper 100, London: Home Office, Policing and Reducing Crime Unit.

Priestley, M. (1999) *Disability Politics and Community Care*, London: Jessica Kingsley.

Radford, L., Sayer, S. and AMICA (1999) *Unreasonable Fears? Child contact in the context of comestic violence: A survey of mothers' perceptions of harm*, Bristol: Women's Aid Publications.

Rai, D. K. and Thiara, R. (1997) *Re-defining Spaces: The needs of black women and children in refuge support services and black workers in women's aid*, Bristol: Women's Aid Federation of England.

Rai, D. K. and Thiara, R. (1999) *Strengthening Diversity: Good practice in delivering domestic violence services to black women and children*, Bristol: Women's Aid Federation of England.

Ramcharan, P., Roberts, G., Grant, G. and Borland, J. (1997) 'Citizenship, empowerment and everyday life: ideal and illusion in the new millennium', in Ramcharan, P., Roberts, G., Grant, G. and Borland, J. (eds) *Empowerment in Everyday Life: Learning disability*, London: Jessica Kingsley.

Rhode, D. L. (1989) *Justice and Gender: Sex discrimination and the law*, Cambridge, MA: Harvard University Press.

Ribbens, J. (1998) 'Hearing my feeling voice?', in Ribbens, J. and Edwards, R. (eds) *Feminist Dilemmas in Qualitative Research*, London: Sage.

Ryan, B. (1992) *Feminism and the Women's Movement: Dynamics of change in social movement ideology and activism*, London: Routledge.

Saunders, H. (2001) *Making Contact Worse? Report of a national survey of domestic violence refuge services into the enforcement of contact orders*, Bristol: Women's Aid Federation of England.

Sayce, L. (1999) *From Psychiatric Patient to Citizen: Overcoming discrimination and social exclusion*, Basingstoke: Macmillan.

Schechter, S. (1982) *Women and Male Violence: The visions and struggles of the battered women's movement*, Boston: South End Press.

Scott, A. (1990) *Ideology and New Social Movements*, London: Unwin Hyman.

Scott, J. (ed.) (1994) *Power: Critical concepts*, London: Routledge.

Scottish Women's Aid (1998) *Young People Say*, Edinburgh: Scottish Women's Aid.

Servian, R. (1996) *Theorising Empowerment: Individual power and community care*, Bristol: The Policy Press.

Shakespeare, T. (1993) 'Disabled people's self-organisation: a new social movement?', *Disability, Handicap and Society* 8(3): 249–64.

Shaping Our Lives (undated) *The Outcomes We Want and How We Can Achieve Them*, leaflet, London: National Institute for Social Work.

Sheridan, A. (1980) *Michel Foucault: The will to truth*, London: Tavistock.

Sissons, P. (1999) *Focus on Change: Report on consultation carried out with women survivors of domestic violence*, London: Lewisham Domestic Violence Forum.

Smith, L. (1989) *Domestic Violence: An overview of the literature*, Home Office Research Study 107, London: Home Office.

Social Care Institute for Excellence (2002) *SCIE: Social Care Institute for Excellence*, leaflet, London: SCIE.

Southall Black Sisters (1990) *Against the Grain: A celebration of survival and struggle*, London: Southall Black Sisters.

Southall Black Sisters (2000) *Southall Black Sisters: Annual report*, London: Southall Black Sisters.

Squires, J. and Kemp, J. (1997) *Feminisms*, Oxford: Oxford University Press.

Stacey, J. (1993) 'Untangling feminist theory', in Richardson, D. and Robinson, V. (eds) *Introducing Women's Studies*, Basingstoke: Macmillan, pp. 49–73.

Standing Together against Domestic Violence (2002) *Survivors Speak: A report on the findings of consultations with survivors of domestic violence 2001–2002*, London: Standing Together.

Stanko, E. A., (2003) *The Meanings of Violence*, London: Routledge.

Stanko, E. A., Crisp, D., Hale, C. and Lucraft, H. (1998) *Counting the Costs: Estimating the impact of domestic violence in the London Borough of Hackney*, London: Crime Concern.

Stanley, L. and Wise, S. (1983) *Breaking Out: Feminist consciousness and feminist research*, London: Routledge and Kegan Paul.

Stanley, L. and Wise, S. (1993) *Breaking Out Again: Feminist ontology and epistemology*, London: Routledge and Kegan Paul.

Stewart, M. and Taylor, M. (1996) *Empowerment and Estate Regeneration*, Bristol: The Policy Press.

Swain, J., Finkelstein, V., Oliver, M. and French, S. (eds) (1993) *Disabling Barriers – Enabling Environments*, London: Sage.

Taylor-Browne, J. (ed.) (2001) *What Works in Reducing Domestic Violence? A comprehensive guide for professionals*, London: Whiting and Birch.

Tutty, L. M., Bidgood, B. A. and Rothery, M. A. (1993) 'Support groups for battered women: research on their efficacy', *Journal of Family Violence* 8: 325–43.

UNICEF (1997) *The Progress of Nations*, New York: UNICEF.

United Nations (1995) *Beijing Declaration and Platform for Global Action, Adopted by the Fourth World Conference on Women, Beijing*, New York: United Nations.

User-Centred Services Group (1993) *Building Bridges Between People Who Use and People Who Provide Services*, London: National Institute for Social Work.

Violence Against Lesbians in the Home (1998) *Lesbians' Own Accounts*, JJ Publications. (Place of publication not cited.)

Walker, L. E. A. (1977–8) 'Battered women and learned helplessness', *Victimology* 2(3/4): 525–34.

Wallerstein, N. (1992) 'Powerlessness, empowerment and health: implications for health promotion programs', *American Journal of Health Promotion* 6(3): 197–205.

Welsh Office (1983) *All Wales Strategy for the Development of Services for Mentally Handicapped People* [*sic*], Cardiff: Welsh Office.

Williams, F. (1992) 'Somewhere over the rainbow: universality and diversity in social policy', in Manning, N. and Page, R. (eds) *Social Policy Review* 4: 200–19.

Williams, F. (1996) 'Postmodernism, feminism and the question of difference', in Parton, N. (ed.) *Social Theory, Social Change and Social Work*, London: Routledge.

Williams, O. (2003) 'Developing the capacity to address social context issues: group treatment with African American men who batter', in Cohen, M. B. and Mullender, A. (eds) *Gender and Groupwork*, London: Routledge.

Williamson, E. (2000) *Domestic Violence and Health: The response of the medical profession*, Bristol: The Policy Press.

Wolf, N. (1993) *Fire with Fire*, London: Chatto and Windus.

Woman Abuse Council of Toronto (1999) *Finding Our Voice: Healing thoughts from survivors of woman abuse*, Toronto: Woman Abuse Council.

Women's Aid Federation of England (1989) *Breaking Through: Women surviving male violence*, Bristol: Women's Aid Federation of England.

Women's Aid Federation of England (1998) *Families Without Fear: Women's Aid agenda for a national strategy*, Bristol: Women's Aid Federation of England.

Women's Aid Federation of England (2001–2) *Women's Aid Annual Report*, Bristol: Women's Aid Federation of England.

Index

Abrahams, H. 83
Abused Women's Perspectives project 3;
    commitment of services to user
    involvement 61, 62–73; and funding 29,
    103; innovatory practice 113, 115;
    practicalities of consultation 93, 95,
    103, 104–8; user involvement 16, 26,
    30, 83, 84, 85, 132, 133, 139, 141–2,
    145, 146; women's views 43, 55–7,
    151–9
activist movement 1, 4, 20, 40, 44–6, 62,
    70, 83, 108, 112, 128, 144, 145, 147;
    early history 7–9; as new social
    movement 9–13; see also refuges;
    Women's Aid; women's organisations
advisory work 4, 50, 112, 113–24, 128,
    142, 147
advocacy 16, 23, 24, 158
advocacy organisations 33, 44, 57, 62, 94,
    96, 97, 99, 103, 128, 130, 133, 140,
    143; innovatory practice 125, 129, 147;
    women's views 63, 68, 73, 158
African Caribbean women 66
African-centred theory 17
ageing see older people
Ahluwalia, Kiranjit 129
All Party Parliamentary Group on
    Domestic Violence 136, 151, 160–2
All Wales Strategy for the Development
    of Services for Mentally Handicapped
    People 32
Ambassador One Stop Project 67
Anderson, J. 29
Arabic-speaking women 66
Area Child Protection Committees
    (ACPCs) 66
Aris, Rosemary 3, 80

Asian women 45, 51, 66, 100, 129, 135,
    153
Asian Women's Resource Centre 100,
    128, 135
asylum seekers 133
Australia 38

Baistow, K. 29
Barnes, M. 94, 96, 100, 120
Batsleer, J. 49, 51
BBC 136
benefits 157, 162
Benefits Agency 56, 158
Beresford, Peter 13, 14, 17, 22, 27, 28, 31,
    33–4, 35
Best Value Framework 23, 92, 147
Binney, V. 46, 52
bisexuals 49
black men, and relational power 37
black women: innovatory practice 128;
    user involvement 32, 33, 39, 66, 100,
    106, 110, 117, 131, 133, 135, 138;
    views on services 20, 48–9, 50, 51
Boal, Agusto 129
Braye, S. 14–15
Brent 100, 128, 135
British Council of Disabled People 96
bureaucracy 28–9, 31, 91, 94, 106, 115

Cabinet Office 161; Women's Unit 47
campaigning 9, 10, 45, 125, 128–30,
    141–2, 147
Campbell, B. 9
Campbell, J. 33–4
Campbell, P. 39
Canada: innovatory practice 123–4;
    refuges 8

Charles, N. 11, 13
Cheshire Domestic Violence Outreach
    Service 47
child-centred research 18
children 145; consultation 48, 136, 138;
    contact arrangements 36, 161, 162;
    decision-making role 72; protection
    20–1, 24, 45, 52, 59; theory 18; views
    on outreach services 57
Children Act (1989) 161
Children and Young People's Strategic
    Partnerships 93
Children's Services Plans 21
Chiswick Women's Aid 8, 9
Citizen's Charter 23, 27
civil justice system 18, 56
class 8, 10, 13, 14, 85, 94
collective advocacy 16, 33
collective empowerment 27, 83, 84–5, 86,
    108, 114, 130; Women's Aid 159
collective organisation 12–13, 23, 27, 31,
    33, 34, 39, 63, 72
community action 33, 79, 129–30
community arts projects 129–30, 147
community care 27, 28, 31, 59
Community Care Plans 21, 23, 93
community development 59, 124
community drop-in centres 118
Community Strategies 93
confidentiality 19, 20, 23, 24; consultation
    and 94, 98, 102, 135; electronic
    consultation 135; user involvement
    79, 85, 120, 132, 133, 134, 146;
    women's views 53, 155, 158
consciousness-raising 8, 10, 16, 26
Conservative governments 27, 28
consultation 27, 34, 145–6; difficulties
    involved in individual survivors
    attending meetings 104–6; electronic
    68, 135–6, 143, 147, 160–2; funding
    and resources 100–3; innovatory
    practice 109–12, 113, 116, 130; need
    for sound policies 94–6; optimum
    methods 142–3; practical issues for
    creating effectiveness 89–108;
    representativeness of domestic violence
    survivors 98–100; translation into
    action 65, 95, 146; user involvement
    28, 31, 50, 52, 59–60, 65–6, 67–8, 69,
    72, 77–88, 110, 133, 134, 135, 136,
    139, 145, 146, 148; Women's Aid and

other women's organisations 125,
    126–8, 130, 155; women's focus groups
    131
consumerist model 23, 24, 27, 28, 94;
    collective, of new social movements 10
Coote, A. 9
Crime and Disorder Act (1998) 92
Crime and Disorder Audits and Strategies
    21, 92, 118, 147
Crime and Disorder Partnerships 92, 97,
    132, 135
criminal justice system 18, 22, 45, 51, 56,
    97, 124, 158, 162
Croft, Suzy 13, 14, 17, 22, 27, 28, 31, 35
Croydon: consultation 92; innovatory
    practice 113–16; One stop shops 67
Croydon Domestic Violence Survivors'
    Forum 79, 113–16
Croydon Empowerment Project 114
Croydon One Stop Partnership 67, 114,
    140–1
culture 85, 94, 102, 117, 133–4, 158

deaf women 49, 134
Dear, Wendy 3
democracy 7, 27
Department of Health 22, 52, 101
developing countries 130
difference 25, 38, 40, 63, 85, 94, 102,
    117; see also diversity
disability 137; social model of 16, 17
disability movement 2, 13, 14, 15, 17, 18,
    20, 58, 81, 96
disabled women 39, 49, 50, 100, 102,
    134, 135
diversity 25, 38, 40, 63, 122, 146;
    inadequate services 48–50; and
    representativeness 99–100; see also
    difference
Dobash, R. E. 46
Dobash, R. P. 22
Domestic Abuse Intervention Project,
    Duluth, Minnesota 109, 124
domestic violence: definition 1; incidence
    in UK 2, 9
Domestic Violence and Minoritisation
    (Batsleer) 49, 51
Domestic Violence Bill 54
domestic violence forums 3, 4, 30, 45,
    60–1; good practice in consultation
    103, 106–7; optimum methods 142;

protocols for user involvement 95, 137–8; user involvement 32, 40, 61–8, 69, 79, 86, 90, 97, 106–8, 133, 137, 143, 145–6, 147, 158; women's organisations and Women's Aid 125, 126, 127, 128
domestic violence survivors 1, 2–3, 4; autonomy 16–17; becoming empowered 18 (see also empowerment); celebration 122; collective organisation 12–13; desired improvements 53–4, 158–9, 162; differences from members of other user movements 19–20, 24; disadvantages of not being regarded as a user movement 22–4; economic problems 12, 94, 157, 162; gaining a voice 16, 24, 26, 44, 58, 125; generating theory 18; identity 81–2, 85; individual participation 104–6, 137, 146; opinions on women's needs 157–8; as professionals 19, 64, 72, 82, 86–7, 142, 143–4, 147, 154; psychological barriers to involvement 32, 94; rejection of negative labels 15–16; representativeness and accountability 33–4, 98–100, 119, 138, 146; self-esteem 83, 84, 85, 94, 101, 119, 138, 154; as service users 7–25; silencing and stigmatisation 19, 20, 24, 47, 74, 80–3, 94, 117, 143–4, 145, 146, 147, 155; training 87, 102, 106, 152–3, 159; views on services 43–57, 151–9; see also user involvement
domestic violence survivors' forums 79, 112, 113–24, 142, 147; key issues 119–24
Dominy, N. 52
Dowson, S. 30, 34
drama 129–30, 147
Dullea, K. 17–18

Economic and Social Research Council: Children 5–16 Years Research Programme 48; Violence Research Programme 3, 43
economic issues 12, 94, 157, 162
e-democracy 160
educational work 45, 106, 117, 158; see also public awareness
electronic consultation 68, 135–6, 143, 147, 160–2

emancipatory 8, 27, 35, 38, 119, 148
empowerment 18, 24, 58, 152, 153; activist movement 16, 44, 70, 108, 130, 159; conflicting models 26–8; obstacles to 26–40, 82, 98; professionalisation of 29–31, 70, 159; user involvement 31, 59, 61, 62, 69–70, 73, 83–6, 90, 109, 142, 146, 147; women's movement 44
environment 11
equality issues 8, 49, 102, 119, 122, 156
Eschle, C. 11
ethnicity 85, 137; see also minority ethnic communities, women from; racism

facilitation 107, 110–11, 122–3, 132, 137
Families Without Fear (Women's Aid) 161
feminism 2, 7, 8, 10, 11, 12, 15, 17–18, 44, 83, 96; and power 35, 36, 38, 40; see also Women's Liberation Movement/women's movement
focus groups 33, 131; women's 65, 112, 131–2, 142–3, 147
forced marriages 161
Foucault, Michel 37–8, 39
funding 46, 59, 100–3, 146, 152, 153, 158; innovatory practice 110, 114, 115, 120, 123; women's focus groups 132; women's organisations 4, 9, 29, 45, 49, 57, 70, 92, 127, 128, 161, 162

gay and lesbian relationships 1; see also lesbians
gender, NSM theory 12
gender discrimination 2, 8; user involvement 33
Gillman, M. 29
Goffman, Erving 31, 81–2
Gondolf, E. 22
good practice 50, 103, 113, 139, 146; electronic consultation 161; excerpts from interviews 156–7
government policy 23, 24, 27, 28, 47, 53, 54; and consultation 91–3; electronic consultation with survivors 160–2
grand theories 38
Grant, G. 31, 32
Grant, W. 10
Greenwich Asian Women's Project 135
Grotberg, E. 84

Hague, Gill 3, 43, 50, 53, 54, 63, 126, 128
Hammersmith, Standing Together against
    Domestic Violence 109–11, 113
Hansard Society 136, 151, 160
Harding, S. 38
Harding, T. 32
Haringey 92
Harwin, Nicola 128, 136; report on
    Womenspeak Internet consultation
    160–2
Health Improvement Programmes
    (HImPs) 23, 93
health services 23, 45; user involvement
    59, 92–3, 97, women's views on 52, 56
helplines 4, 44, 157, 158, 159, 161
Henderson, S. 50, 51, 53
Home Office 92, 128; Briefing Notes
    43–4, 47; Crime Reduction Programme
    on Violence against Women 47, 67,
    141
homophobia 11, 49, 50
homosexual relationships 1; see also
    lesbians
housing 44, 52–3, 56, 57, 59, 67, 92, 157,
    162
Humphreys, Cathy 50, 52, 54–5, 56–7, 72,
    135, 162
Humphreys, Emma 129

identity 10, 13–14, 31, 81–2, 85
Imkaan 45, 129
immigrant women 45, 85, 162; see also
    minority ethnic communities, women
    from
immigration law 161
information 9, 50, 158, 162
inter-agency initiatives see multi-agency
    initiatives
international activism 130, 143
Internet 68, 135–6, 143, 147, 160–2
Irish women travellers 160–1

James-Hanman, D. 48, 128, 135

Kaur, Balwant 129
Kelly, Liz 16, 51–2, 56

labelling 119; rejection of negative 15–16
language issues 102, 121, 132, 133, 158
law: requirement of user involvement 59;
    user involvement in work on use of 117

learning difficulties, people with 17, 23,
    30, 147; services for women 51
legislation 52, 91–3, 128, 162; and
    housing 52–3
'Legislative Theatre' groups 129–30
lesbian theory 17
lesbians 32, 39, 49, 50, 134
Lewisham 50
Lindow, V. 34
Liverpool Domestic Violence Forum 118,
    138
Liverpool, innovatory methods 116,
    118–19
Living Without Fear (Cabinet Office)
    161
local authorities 22, 45, 53; and
    consultation 50, 91–3, 97, 132;
    innovatory practice 114–16; see also
    social services; social work
Local Government Act (2000) 93
London: special mechanisms for user
    involvement 133, 135; see also Brent;
    Croydon; Hammersmith; Haringey;
    Lewisham; Newham; Westminster
Lukes, S. 35–6
Luton, electronic consultation 160–1

Making Research Count 135
Malos, E. 50, 53, 54
Mama, Amina 48, 51, 54
managerialism 28–9, 34
market research 33
Maynard, M. 23
mental health service users 29–30, 95–6;
    see also psychiatric survivors
mentoring 102
Metropolitan Police, Community Safety
    Unit 100
migrant women see immigrant women
minority ethnic communities, women
    from 45; empowerment 84, 85;
    innovatory practice 128, 129; user
    involvement 33, 39, 106, 110, 117, 131,
    133–4, 138; women's views
    48–9, 51, 54, 153, 162; see also black
    women
modernisation agenda 28
Moran, Margaret 160
Morley, R. 53
Mullender, Audrey 3, 17–18, 21, 40, 43,
    50, 52, 53

multi-agency initiatives 39, 53–4;
  innovatory practice in Hammersmith
  109–11; women's focus groups 131;
  see also domestic violence forums

National Health Service see health
  services
National User Involvement Project 22
National Women's Aid Federation 9
National Women's Liberation Conference
  (1978) 8
networking 10, 92
Newcastle 130
Newham, women's focus groups 131
New Labour 28
New Right 27, 28
new social movements 2, 7, 33, 59; as
  forerunners of service user movements
  13–14; neglect of female contribution
  in NSM theory 11–13, 24; women's
  movement as 9–11
NHS see health services
NHS and Community Care Act (1990)
  93
Northern Ireland Women's Aid 9
NVQ courses 87

older people 14, 18; women 15, 39
Oldman, H. 32
Oliver, M. 13
One stop shops 67, 159
Open Service Project 22
outreach services 4, 44, 50; user
  involvement 68–72, 125, 143; women's
  views 56–7, 158, 162

Pahl, J. 52
partnerships 50, 63, 92, 93, 125, 132, 135,
  142
patriarchy 35, 37, 38
peace movement 11
perpetrator programmes 22, 62, 117, 124,
  138, 145
personal and political 11, 12, 13, 15, 39
Phoenix Group 77, 106–7, 116–17
Pizzey, Erin 9
police 45, 50; consultation 100, 106; user
  involvement 67, 97; women's views
  51–2, 55, 56, 157, 158
policy 4, 145; contribution of Women's
  Aid and women's organisations 125,

127, 128, 142–3; difficulties of
  individual survivors attending meetings
  104–6; effective development 136–9;
  innovatory practice 113, 116, 117, 118,
  119, 122, 124, 130; optimum methods
  142–3; user involvement 2, 43, 47, 50,
  59–60, 62, 64, 65, 66, 69, 84, 86–8,
  94–6, 100, 108, 136–9, 140, 144, 146,
  148, 157; women's focus groups 131;
  women's views 68, 151–2, 159
politics 10, 13–14
postcolonial theory 17
postmodernism 34, 37, 39, 63
post-structuralism 37, 39
poverty 94
power 28, 29, 30, 34–9, 40; and
  consultation 89–90; as domination
  35–6; relational 37–9; user involvement
  63–4, 65, 69, 72, 78, 105, 112, 124,
  125, 136, 146, 147; see also
  empowerment
practice 4, 145; critical 38; protocols 95,
  110, 137–8, 146; see also good practice
prevention work 106, 117, 138
Priestley, M. 17
professionals and professionalism:
  consultation 94, 105; and
  empowerment/power 29–31, 33, 39, 70,
  159; excerpts from interviews 152–4,
  156, 157; survivors as 19, 64, 72, 82,
  86–7, 142, 143–4, 147, 154; and user
  involvement 61, 70–1, 78, 86–7, 115,
  121; women's views 50
psychiatric survivors 13, 14, 15, 18, 19,
  20, 58
public awareness 9, 117, 118, 129, 138,
  141–2
public meetings 92, 133

Quality Protects guidance 23
queer theory 17
questionnaires 112, 134–5, 142, 147, 158

racism 11, 32, 37, 48, 49, 51, 102, 134,
  156
Radford, L. 52
radical feminists 8
Rai, D. K. 49, 51
rape 129, 130
rape crisis centres 20
Refuge 9

refugees 66, 133
refuges 4, 20; children's role 48;
  collective motivation 13; and
  consultation 92, 97, 160; early
  organisation 8–9, 10, 36, 44;
  empowerment 16, 83; innovatory
  practice 125–8; representativeness 99;
  training for service users 87; user
  involvement 40, 45, 62, 67, 68–72, 119,
  133, 143; women's views 49, 50, 51,
  53, 56–7, 158, 161, 162; see also
  Women's Aid
Research in Practice 135
research projects 127, 128, 134–5
resistance 34, 37, 39, 40
resource mobilisation theory (RMT) 12
revolutionary feminists 8
Rhode, D. L. 38
Routes to Safety (Humphreys and Thiara)
  54–5, 56–7, 135, 162

safe houses see refuges
safety 19, 146; electronic consultation
  135–6; user involvement 23, 79, 85, 94,
  96, 98, 102, 110, 120, 132, 133, 134,
  146; women's views 2, 50, 53, 57, 60,
  146, 155, 158, 159
Scotland: domestic violence 22; women's
  views on services 50
Scottish Women's Aid 9, 48
second-wave feminism see Women's
  Liberation Movement/women's
  movement
self-advocacy 16, 60, 123, 140
self-help 21, 99, 140
Servian, R. 31, 32, 35
services 3; accountability 4, 16, 59, 60,
  61, 78, 79, 80, 90, 95–6, 112, 124, 133,
  147, 148, 162; benefits of listening to
  women 21–2, 25; extent of commitment
  to user involvement 58–74; optimum
  methods 142–3; participation of
  domestic violence survivors see user
  involvement; respect for survivors 52,
  107, 110, 111; women's views 43–57,
  117, 158–9; see also good practice;
  user movements
sexism 35
sexual assault, services for women 51
sexuality 137, 156
Shakespeare, T. 13

Shaping Our Lives disability project 18
shelters see refuges
Sheridan, A. 37
Social Care Institute for Excellence
  (SCIE) 23, 135
social class see class
social inclusion and exclusion 25, 89
socialism 7, 39
socialist feminists 8
social justice 7
social policy 45
social services 22; women's views 52, 56,
  157
social work 20–1, 23–4, 45, 87
Southall Black Sisters 45, 48, 129
spoiled identity 31, 81–2
standpoint approaches 39
statutory agencies 4, 20; excerpts from
  interviews 153–4; exploitation of
  survivors 118; optimum methods
  142–3; user involvement 40, 61–8,
  70, 73, 103, 108, 140, 142, 143, 145;
  women's views 46–7, 56
structuralism 39
subjectivities 38
Supporting People programme 57, 92,
  128, 161
surveys 92, 112, 127, 134–5, 142, 147
survivors' forums 79, 112, 113–24, 142,
  147; key issues 119–24

Thatcherism 27, 28
'Theatre of the Oppressed' movement
  129–30
Them Wifeys 130
Thiara, R. 49, 51, 54–5, 56–7, 135, 162
Thornton, Sara 129
tokenism 24, 29, 33, 40, 89
Toronto, refuges 8
Toronto Woman Abuse Council 123–4
travellers 160–1
Tutty, L. M. 51

United Nations 130
United States: electronic consultation 135;
  multi-agency projects 109, 124; refuges
  8; reporting abuse 22; support groups
  51
University of Warwick, Centre for the
  Study of Safety and Well-being 54, 135
User-Centred Services Group 22

user control 2, 16–17, 27, 31, 34, 40, 63, 95, 130, 140, 146
user involvement 2, 4, 16, 24, 26, 88, 139–42, 144, 145–8; attitudes to being 'in the experience' 3, 73–4, 85, 143–4; barriers to 31–4; basic initial checklist 97; benefits of listening to women 21–2, 25; excerpts from interviews 151–9; gendered hierarchy 33; good practice 50, 103, 113, 139, 146, 156–7; innovatory practice 109–24, 146–7; key issues 96, 98–100; in multi-agency forums and statutory agencies 61–8; and power 34–9, 89–90; reasons for 58–61; representativeness and accountability 33–4, 98–100, 119, 138, 146; special mechanisms 132–4; women's refuge, support and outreach services 68–72; see also consultation; professionals and professionalism
user movements 1–2, 39, 59, 63, 94; absence of women 2, 14–15, 24, 43; accountability 95–6, 98; differences between abused women and others 19–20; disadvantages to abused women of being disregarded 22–4; new social movements as forerunners 13–14; reasons for absence of women 20–1; resemblances between aims and those of women's movement 15–18

Valuing People White Paper 23
Violence Against Lesbians in the Home 51
Voice for Change 116, 118–19

Walker, L. E. A. 16
Wearside Women in Need project 141
Welsh Women's Aid 9
Westminster Domestic Violence Forum 103, 106–7, 116
Westminster, innovatory methods 116–17
Williams, F. 14, 23

Women and Equality Unit 47
Women's Aid 4, 45, 47; children's role 48; early organisation 8–9, 10; electronic consultation 136, 151, 160, 161; empowerment 83; innovatory practice 125–30, 147; user involvement 21, 63, 65, 68, 70–2, 102, 112, 135, 141, 142, 147, 155; women's views 50, 51, 54, 155, 159; see also refuges
Women's Aid Federation of England 4, 9, 87, 151, 161
Women's Aid National Agenda for Action 161
women's focus groups 65, 112, 131–2, 142–3, 147
Women's Liberation Movement/women's movement 2, 37–8, 112; early activism 7–9, 36; as a new social movement 9–11, 12; resemblances between aims and those of user movements 15–18, 24; see also activist movement
women's organisations 3, 4, 20, 44–5, 132, 140, 145–6; empowerment 83; innovatory practice 125–30, 147; women's views 50–1; see also advocacy organisations; outreach services; Women's Aid; women's support organisations
Womenspeak 160–2; summary of findings 162
women's support organisations 44, 45, 50–1, 57, 62; and consultation 92, 96, 97, 99; and empowerment 83–4; user involvement 62, 68–72, 73, 113, 129, 133, 143, 147; women's views 49, 57, 158, 159
Women's Unit of the Cabinet Office 47

Young People Say (Scottish Women's Aid) 48
young women: innovatory practice 130; services for 51

Lightning Source UK Ltd.
Milton Keynes UK
UKOW05f1804311016
286565UK00018B/615/P

9 780415 259460